ACTION MOVIE HERO WORKOUTS

GET SUPER CRIME FIGHTER RIPPED

DAVE RANDOLPH

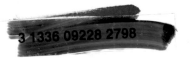

Published in the United States by
Ulysses Press
P.O. Box 3440
Berkeley, CA 94703
www.ulyssespress.com

ISBN: 978-1-61243-063-8
Library of Congress Control Number 2012937120

Printed in the United States by Bang Printing

10 9 8 7 6 5 4 3 2 1

Acquisitions: Keith Riegert
Managing editor: Claire Chun
Editor: Lily Chou
Proofreader: Elyce Berrigan-Dunlop
Production: Jake Flaherty
Index: Sayre Van Young
Cover design: what!design @ whatweb.com
Cover photographs: background © Mikhail/shutterstock.com; man © dpaint/shutterstock.com
Models: Michael Espero, Meredith Miller, Dave Randolph, Brett Stewart

CONTENTS

PART 1: OVERVIEW

INTRODUCTION

When you were a kid, maybe you tied a bedsheet around your neck and tore through the house pretending you were Superman, Batman or Supergirl. Or maybe you donned a mask and karate-chopped and kicked your way through hundreds of imaginary bad guys as Kato from *The Green Hornet*. As an adult, you can absolutely get that smoking-hot physique your favorite action hero is known for.

Action Movie Hero Workouts features easy-to-follow exercise programs that anyone can do to sculpt their bodies into blockbuster shape. Although the actual workouts the actors in this book used to get their trademark looks are a closely guarded secret, we examined the few we did find and used our decades of fitness-training experience to create programs that will get you the physique you want.

Don't fall for the "patented" quick fat-loss secrets of the stars—nutrition and hard work are all it takes and all that works. We show you how to add muscle mass like Chris Evans and Chris Hemsworth. We teach you how to get lean and ripped like Robert Downey Jr. in *Sherlock Holmes* and Brad Pitt in *Fight Club*.

You may notice that Jessica Biel is the only female action star in this book. It's not because there's a lack of strong female

loads—it's simply because female action stars often share the same physique and likely do similar if not identical workouts. In fact, many shared the same trainer. While all these women look great, they don't necessarily have defined arms and shoulders, a shapely rear end or killer thighs that can kick some serious butt. Biel fits the bill as a bonafide action hero, not just a pretty face with a model's body.

Whether you want to look like Thor, Captain America, James Bond or Lara Croft, *Action Movie Hero Workouts* will help you develop your action-hero body of choice with exercise programs and advice on nutrition. With hard work, the dedication to follow the programs to a T and, most importantly, diet, you'll bulk up your slender figure or transform your overweight self into a lean, ripped machine.

HOW TO USE THIS BOOK

Getting an action-hero physique requires a few simple things: reading this book (including the nutrition section), studying the exercises, and getting off the couch. If you aren't already vigorously exercising on a regular basis, please get the okay to begin from your doctor. The workouts in this book can be very demanding and you need to make sure your body can handle the stress.

You'll then want to decide which action hero you'd like to look like. Once you've made your choice, dig into the training program for that action hero and determine what kind of equipment you'll need. Follow the program as written—make no modifications unless you have a pre-existing condition that prohibits you from doing certain exercises. Make sure you warm up beforehand (see pages 138–40 for suggestions)! Doing so prepares your body for the work you're about to do.

We've tried to include progressions/regressions wherever possible to make it easier or harder based on your ability to do a movement. For example, here's the progression for lunges:

Level 1–Static Lunge/Split Squat Hold

Level 2–Static Lunge/Split Squat rise up and down

Level 3–Forward Lunge

Level 4–Reverse Lunge

Level 5–Walking Lunge

Level 6–Jumping Lunge

Each level requires specific skills, so if you haven't mastered level 3, you shouldn't be doing level 6. It's a safety issue.

Make sure your technique is as close to perfect as you can get—practice the movement. Don't get hung up on trying to go too heavy or as quickly as you can. Both lead to poor form and increase the potential for injury.

Exercise Terms

There's a lot of jargon and abbreviations used in the exercise world. We define some of the terms here so you'll know what they mean and how to use them when you read the workouts.

Repetition, or rep: The number of times you do an exercise.

Set: A specific number of reps for one exercise. You'll typically see "5x5," "5x8," etc., where the first number is the total number of sets and the second is the number of reps per set. Thus you have 5 sets of 5 reps, 5 sets of 8 reps. You may also see "8x5" or "5x3." This is still sets and reps: 8 sets of 5 reps, 5 sets of 3 reps. Note that 5x8 and 8x5 are the same total reps (i.e., 40) but the first should be done with a lighter weight than the second. Typically the lower the number of reps, the heavier the weight.

Superset: Doing 2 different exercises one right after the other, usually with little to no rest. This is typically written as "1a) Deadlift 1b) Pull-ups." This means you'll do the prescribed number of reps for the deadlift followed immediately by the prescribed number of pull-ups. Then you'll go back to the deadlift. The sets are almost always the same:

1a) Deadlift 3x6

1b) Pull-Ups 3xAMRAP

2a) Bench Press 3x10

2b) Curls 3x6

That's 6 deadlifts, then as many reps as possible (AMRAP) of pull-ups, then repeat 2 more times. The 2a) 2b) pairing indicates a second superset. You'll usually have a few minutes of rest between the supersets. Note that some trainers also write them as "A1) A2)."

Tri-set: Doing 3 exercises back to back, or 1a) 1b) 1c). This works the same as the superset.

Circuit: More than 3 exercises performed back to back. You cycle through all the exercises in the circuit, doing all prescribed reps for all exercises back to back before repeating the first exercise.

Rest Period: The amount of rest between exercises or sets. Sometimes there'll be rest between exercises, especially in a high-intensity interval training (HIIT) circuit; other times there may be rest after the last exercise of a super- or tri-set before you repeat it. There's almost always rest at the end of a super- or tri-set before going to the next grouping. Try to stick to the rest, especially if you're out of shape. Taking too long allows the heart rate to drop too low (under 130 to 140 beats per minute), which slows down the fat-burning process. If you're in fairly good shape and find the rest periods too long, by all means shorten them, but not so much that you can't complete the next exercise.

Time: Some exercises, supersets, etc., are done based on time rather than reps. This is typical of a HIIT circuit. The goal is to use a weight that's challenging to you but still allows you to work the entire time period (typically 20 or 30 seconds). When you see "20" in the Time column and "10" in the Rest column, that means hit it as hard as you can for the time, then rest the amount of time allotted in the rest column. The shorter the work period, the faster you should go! Crank it and try to maintain that pace. This

is especially true of bodyweight exercises like mountain climbers, squat thrusts and burpees. These circuits are generally used as "finishers" at the end of the workout.

Time Under Tension, or TUT: The pace you should do each part of the movement. For example, you might see "3-1-2" for a biceps curl. The first number is the first part of the movement (depending on the movement it could be a contraction or an extension), the second number is the pause, while the third number is the return to the start position:

- Count to 3 as the dumbbells come closer to your chest.

- Pause for 1 count with the biceps fully contracted.

- Count to 2 as you return the weight back to the start position.

Doing reps this way will make you a lot stronger without necessarily using a ton of weight. You'll only see TUT numbers on "grinding" exercises—those that aren't inherently done quickly, like a barbell clean

CHART ABBREVIATIONS

AMRAP	As Many Reps as Possible
KB	Kettlebell
DB	Dumbbell
BB	Barbell
R/L	Do the given number of reps on the right side, then switch to the left.
L1/L2/L3	Level 1/Level 2/Level 3
H2H	Hand to Hand
HIIT	High-Intensity Interval Training

BUILDING MUSCLE

Ladies, this is directed toward you but applies to the guys as well: Lift heavy or go home! That means you should be lifting as heavy as you can, appropriate to the exercise, sets, reps and time you're dealing with. Doing 10 barbell deadlifts with 15 pounds is great if you're six years old or doing rehab exercise, but for an adult female it's nonsense. Lifting heavy builds strong, dense muscle. If you do the programs in this book, you won't look like a bodybuilder—you'll look like Jessica, or fairly close (not the guys, though).

or a kettlebell swing. For grinding exercises where we don't specify a TUT, be reasonable and find a moderate pace. Don't just toss the weight around; if you can, it's too light.

Gear

You'll need some basic equipment to whip your body into action-hero shape. Most programs require a barbell and dumbbells, and perhaps a kettlebell or 2. The Jessica Biel workout also requires resistance bands that have 10–15 or 15–30 pounds resistance, possibly heavier. Three pairs of bands will generally do the trick.

You may also need a stability ball, access to a squat rack or stand, and a bench for bench presses (one that can be adjusted is best). Optional equipment include a wheelbarrow, heavy ropes, a sledgehammer, a big tire, a pushing/pulling sled, a Roman chair and a glute/hamstring raise.

Once you've gathered the equipment or found a facility that has the gear you need, you're ready to start. Post-workout, you may want to invest in a foam roller. Foam rolling is essential to maintaining healthy tissue. Using a foam roller helps reduce soreness, improves blood flow and helps eliminate trigger points. For additional soreness relief, you should also get and use a small ball such as that used for lacrosse (harder, more intense) or tennis (softer, more yielding).

EAT LIKE AN ACTION HERO

Proper eating is essential to developing the lean, chiseled look of an action hero—unless you want to look like Chris Farley in *Beverly Hills Ninja!* Consuming the right amount of protein, good fats and non-starchy carbs will help you build lean muscle mass and strip off body fat.

Most of the action heroes in this book followed typical bodybuilder dietary habits. Generally, they:

- Ate 4–6 small meals throughout the day

- Ate lean protein or had a shake with every meal

- Ate non-starchy carbs (veggies) with every meal

- Ate starchy carbs (like a baked potato or nutritionally dense bread) after high-exertion workouts

- Ate good fats (nuts, avocados, olive or coconut oil, fish oil)

- Avoided alcohol (a drink or two on the weekends was okay, but only one or two)

Those who were bulking up typically ingested about 4000–5000 calories and drank a lot of protein shakes. Those dropping weight ate fewer calories (in the 2500–3500 range) and less protein. No one—not even Jessica Biel—went on a low-calorie (under 1200 calories) diet. If you eat too little you'll lose weight, but it's muscle, not fat. So although your weight will go down, you won't get defined muscles.

Muscle tone and being lean and ripped is solely a function of body fat. You can exercise until the cows come home, but if your body fat percentage stays the same, you'll never have any definition. Bodybuilders in the past (and some still do this) went through phases: bulking and cutting. During the bulking phase they pretty much ate anything that came close enough to put in their mouths. During the cutting phase they decreased their calories and increased their cardio. The problem with this: It isn't sustainable or doable by the average person—you!

It's a common recommendation to eat four to six times per day. Doing so is supposed to keep your insulin levels steady, prevent you from feeling hungry so you don't overeat at your next meal, provide a steady source of fuel, and a host of other things. Bodybuilders have been eating this way for years, but it can be tough to stick to. It requires a lot of planning and preparing food in advance, but if you can do that, it's fantastic. If not, eating three times a day is okay too.

Some people are now trying "intermittent fasting." The idea is that you eat all your daily required calories in a six- to eight-hour window. The rest of the day you eat nothing or very little. You're still getting your caloric requirements for the day, just all at once. The body only knows it needs energy and doesn't care if it comes all at once (filling up the tank when it's on "E") or three to six times per day

(topping off the tank every day). Many people have lost a lot of weight with intermittent fasting and put on tons of muscle at the same time. Do the research, try it for yourself and see what happens.

Here's our dietary advice in a nutshell:

• Not all carbs are bad—get 25% of your calories/day from veggies and fruit.

• Animal-based protein is by far the best for building lean muscle—eat 30–35% of your calories/day from protein.

• Fats are necessary for maintaining healthy skin and joints—consume 40–45% of your daily caloric intake from nuts, avocados, coconut oil, olive oil and naturally occurring fats in meat and poultry, including bacon (but don't go overboard on meat-based fats).

• Eat whole foods—the less processed the better, the longer they (especially grains) take to cook the better.

• Eat raw—try to eat most of your veggies as raw as possible, although some veggies are actually better for you steamed. You'll cook all the vitamins and minerals away if you cook veggies to mush.

• Eat fresh—get your food from a source that's as close to home as possible.

Proteins, Carbs, Fats & Alcohol

A healthy diet should consist of 25% fibrous carbohydrates, followed by 30-35% protein. The rest of your calories should come from good fats. Depending on your specific goals you may need to adjust these numbers slightly. If you're trying to build muscle, increase your protein intake a little and drop the fibrous carbs by the same amount. Don't be afraid of fats—your body needs them for cellular functions as well as energy. Fats have been demonized over the past 30 to 40 years but better modern research is showing that we need fats more than we need carbs.

Protein: Protein is what muscle is made of. When you exercise, no matter what type of exercise, your body actually breaks down muscle (protein) for energy. Lifting heavy also causes microscopic tears in the muscle. The process of breaking down muscle is known as catabolism. In magazines you'll see people talking about being in a catabolic state.

The opposite of that is anabolism. When you're in an anabolic state, you're building muscle. In order to be in an anabolic state you must eat protein. You have to not only replenish what the body used as fuel, you have to eat more than you burned in order to fuel the muscle-building process!

Protein also contains amino acids. Some are essential and some are not. Essential amino acids are those the body requires but cannot make itself, therefore you must get them from food. Protein from meat is the most complete source of amino acids. It has all the essential amino acids as well as those that the body can make for itself. Branched chain amino acids (or BCAAs) are a specific type of amino acid that can provide a huge energy boost.

No matter which eating style you choose, you should always eat protein, be it lean beef, chicken, turkey or fish. It's required if you want to build muscle and get strong.

AVOID SOY

The Chinese have been eating soy for 5000 years or more and written documents from that period show that they ate the roots, not the beans. They knew that unfermented soy was bad for them. Guess what—it still is! Stay away from soy-based proteins (soy protein powder, soy milk) unless they're fermented, Japanese style. Tofu isn't fermented, but items such as miso, natto and tempeh are. Unfermented soy has a lot of estrogenic properties and many doctors will prescribe soy milk instead of estrogen pills to women for hormone replacement therapy (HRT). This means guys could get the dreaded "man-boobs" and decreased testosterone levels.

Hundreds of foods out there are loaded with soybeans since it's used as filler, as a primary protein source and as the main ingredient in almost all vegan/vegetarian meat substitute foods like vegan "burgers." Make sure to read labels before you buy.

We're not fond of pork as a protein source but if you like it, eat it in moderation. If you're a vegetarian, eat a high-quality plant-based protein such as peas or rice. Stay away from soy-based protein. If you eat eggs, eat the whole egg—the yolks are where most of the protein is. Don't be afraid of dietary cholesterol.

If you're on a big mass-building effort and are already eating properly, add a high-quality whey-based protein source to your diet. It should contain protein, branched chain amino acids (BCAAs) and perhaps some vitamins, minerals and flavorings. The sugar content should be low, and there should be absolutely no artificial sweeteners of any kind (e.g., sucralose, maltose, maltitol, high-fructose corn syrup, NutraSweet/aspartame, saccharine).

The good stuff is not cheap, but you get what you pay for. Inexpensive protein is not quality protein and you won't see anywhere near the results. Pay a little, use a lot or pay a lot and use a little; the bottom line is it's much cleaner with no junk added. You may also find that intestinal problems are a fairly common occurrence with lesser-quality proteins.

Carbohydrates: Carbs are an energy source and provide fiber in the diet. Your body also gets vitamins and minerals from carb-based foods so not eating fruits and veggies will lead to lower energy levels and many health issues related to the lack of certain vitamins and minerals. These deficiencies can be seen and felt—everything from muscle cramps (magnesium deficiency), to hair falling out (iron and the amino acid l-lysine), to more frequent and more severe colds (vitamins C and D), to lethargy (B vitamins) and much more. Supplementing with vitamins helps but many vitamins are junk, which is a discussion for another book.

It seems many people are afraid of all carbs these days and even avoid vegetables and fruits because they contain carbs. On one hand "starchy" carbs like white potatoes and grains can wreak havoc on your insulin levels and are now being blamed for the rise in obesity levels over the past 50 years. There's a definite correlation between obesity and the low-fat/high-carb diets that most people are on today.

Grains in the form of breads and pastas are okay in very small quantities but most people eat way too much. Almost all grains contain gluten and some people who are

If you eat right all the time, you increase your muscle mass by lifting heavy weights. The food helps fuel the process. If you eat a lot but lift light, you won't build muscle, only fat.

gluten sensitive may not know it. Crohn's disease and other inflammatory diseases have risen along with obesity and the increase in grain-based foods.

Fibrous carbs (spinach, broccoli, cauliflower, lettuce, kale, carrots, etc.), on the other hand, provide a substantial portion of essential vitamins and minerals and should make up the majority of your diet. You can eat a whole bag of baby carrots and not gain any weight at all. The same goes for a big container of spinach.

Eat all the salad you want, but no bread or croutons. Dressing, if you must have it, should be extra virgin olive oil and a high-quality balsamic vinegar. Stay away from pre-packaged salad dressings, which tend to contain high-fructose corn syrup, soy and possibly artificial sweeteners.

Here are sources of starchy carbs that are okay in moderation:

- Quinoa-based pasta
- Dense bread that's 100% whole grain (if a loaf feels heavy, it probably has more nutrients per slice)—the ingredient list shouldn't have enriched flour of any kind, nor added sugar or molasses
- Legumes, beans and peas have tons of fiber and protein, although fruits and veggies are a better source of fiber and meat is the best source of protein

• Long-grain rice and wild rice, but stay away from white rice—like other grains, the longer it takes to cook, the better it is

• Yams and sweet potatoes, eaten plain or with a bit of real butter

Note that this doesn't mean you can go out and eat starchy carbs at each meal or even every day. Keep your starchy carb intake to an hour or so before or after your workout. Eating them pre-workout will increase your glucose levels, giving you more energy. Eating them post-workout replenishes those glucose stores and actually helps build muscle when ingested in conjunction with lean protein. A baked potato, plain or with real butter, is a great carb source as long as you eat it after a hard workout. Eating potatoes every day, especially loaded with sour cream and all the other junk, will make you fat.

After a workout, especially a tough one, your body craves protein to rebuild muscle and carbs for immediate energy. By taking them together within an hour or so after working out, your body will pull the nutrients into your body more quickly than usual and make them more readily available. The increase in insulin from the carbs helps pull more nutrients into your system right after a workout so you'll get more protein to the muscles. The protein helps stabilize and minimize the insulin spike and the subsequent drop.

The morning is another good time to eat starchy carbs such as steel-cut oatmeal (not the instant kind—the longer it takes to cook, the better it is for you). They help get your brain going and provide some quick energy. If you don't eat protein with it, you're much more likely to crash an hour or so later, unless you're drinking a lot of coffee. At breakfast the protein slows the insulin secretion and keeps you on a more even keel. To get more protein at breakfast, mix in some natural or organic peanut butter, almond butter or even protein powder; do so after the oatmeal has finished cooking to avoid protein breakdown from the heat. You can also mix in fresh berries as well.

In many circles fruit has gotten a bad rap: It's a sugary carb, it'll make you fat. This is B.S. The vitamins and minerals you don't get from veggies you get from fruit, which should be fresh and, wherever possible, organic to avoid pesticides. Sure, fruit is sugar (fructose, to be exact), but your body responds differently to fructose than it does to sucrose (table sugar). Fructose causes a lower insulin response than sucrose.

Fructose is a monosaccharide, while sucrose is a disaccharide (or two molecules, one fructose and one glucose). When you eat fruit, your body can immediately use the fructose for energy or store it as fat. When you eat regular sugar, it gets spilt into glucose and fructose. The glucose triggers a whole cascade of events in the body, including signaling the body to pull excess glucose out of the bloodstream for storage.

All types of sugar can be used immediately for energy. If they aren't burned off, they get stored as fat. Recent studies have shown that it doesn't matter what type of sugar you eat—if you eat too much, it'll make you fat. However, you have to eat 20 apples every day to make any difference in body fat percentage. Twenty apples would equal about 500 calories from sugar; the same holds true for pears. On a 2000-calories-per-day diet, that's 25% of your calories from sugar. Other fruits like berries, oranges and peaches have less fructose so you'd have to eat even more of them to have a significant effect on fat stores.

So should you eat fruit? Yes. An apple or a banana a day, berries in your oatmeal or salad—the benefits are great and you can't possibly eat enough of them to keep you from losing fat. If, however, you're in the last phase of preparing for a bodybuilding contest, you should stop eating fruit, but that's only if you're one of those few who want to be 5–6% body fat. For everyone else, one or two pieces of fruit a day won't make a difference.

Fats: Fats found in lean protein such as lean beef, chicken and turkey, coconut and palm kernel oil, avocados and fresh fish are essential to maintaining healthy skin and joints but you shouldn't consume too much. We typically recommend that 40–45% of your daily caloric intake come from fat, including fish oil supplements.

There are three types of fats: saturated, unsaturated and trans-fats. Saturated fat comes mostly from animal sources (think butter, lard and solid shortening) and many doctors think they're bad for you. The prevalent belief that butter is bad because it has higher levels of cholesterol and saturated fat than margarine is still being pushed by the "health" organizations. New research, however, is showing that butter is much better for you than margarine. We also now see that eating an entire egg isn't bad either. Cholesterol in food doesn't play a role in high cholesterol in the body. High cholesterol in the body is now being viewed as an inflammatory response to stress and sensitivity to all the grains we eat these days.

Unsaturated fat comes in two varieties: mono and poly. Considered "good fats," they're a part of a healthy diet. Mono-unsaturated fats, which are liquid at room temperature but solidify when cold, can be found in olives, olive oil, nuts, peanut oil, canola oil and avocados. Some studies have shown that these kinds of fats can actually lower LDL (bad) cholesterol and maintain HDL (good) cholesterol. Poly-unsaturated fats are also liquid at room temperature and are found in safflower, sesame, corn and other oils. They're thought to lower LDL and raise HDL as well. Trans-fats are man-made and no doubt you've heard about how bad they are; food manufacturers are removing them from their products.

The Atkins diet made low-carb, high-fat diets a huge fad that's still popular but controversial today. Basically it involves avoidance of all carbs, including vegetables, which is nonsense, as explained earlier. Another problem with high-fat-type diets is that people eat the wrong type of fat. Typically they figure they can eat tons of McDonald's burgers because they contain protein and fat, but the wrong kind of fat (saturated) or too much fat in general can cause health problems. Eating a home-cooked sirloin or bison burger is much healthier than a burger from a fast-food joint.

The demonization of meat and, by extension, fats, by the press, vegans, vegetarians and even the American Medical Association and American Heart Association is based on faulty science. Poorly done studies, with intentionally skewed or hidden data by those who may have an agenda, have caused many people to think fat is bad, hence the low-fat fad of the 1970s and '80s. If you look at the incidence of obesity from the '70s on, when food producers were coming out with low-fat everything, obesity has gone up steadily. Replacing fat with artificial fats and adding in sugar and artificial sweeteners made people think they could eat more because their favorite foods had less fat and were therefore okay to eat.

The American Diabetes Association (ADA) and American Heart Association (AHA) continually recommend the use of vegetable oil instead of animal fats. According to several well-done studies, however, the use of vegetable oil may actually cause or increase the likelihood of cancer. Your body must have fat in order to utilize fat-soluble vitamins like A, D, E and K. The problem with eating low fat is that your body

will run out of those vitamins and not be able to utilize them. The fat is required to allow the body to use those vitamins. You don't have to eat the vitamins every day. Your liver stores them if they aren't used, but the supply has to be replenished. The only way to do so is by ingesting fats.

Alcohol: If you're trying to get totally ripped, like 5% body fat, stay away from alcohol. Fermented alcohol, like beer and wine, contains sugar, or carbs. Distilled beverages such as whiskey, vodka and rum don't have any sugar but most people mix in sugary flavorings (margaritas, anyone?), which is where the vast majority of calories comes from. With seven calories per gram, it actually contains more calories than protein and carbs. Only fat, coming in at nine, has more calories per gram. Protein and carbs both contain four calories per gram.

If you're trying to get lean (say, in the 10–15% body fat range), a few beers or a glass of wine on the weekends isn't going to make much of a difference. However, you should avoid mixed drinks completely. The mixtures are typically loaded with sugar, which you should be making every effort to stay away from. If you must drink a cocktail, try mixing it with 10% natural fruit juice (not from concentrate). Margaritas and other mixes will pack on the pounds very quickly.

PART 2: PROGRAMS

CHRISTIAN BALE
WORKOUT APPROACH FOR
BATMAN—THE DARK KNIGHT

Christian Bale, probably the best Batman to date, transformed himself from a scrawny 120 pounds (some say 130) to a brawny 220 or 230. What's impressive is that his 100-pound weight gain was almost all muscle and he did it in six months! Most coaches will tell you it's impossible to put on that much muscle mass in such a short time without the use of steroids. On average he would've gained almost 17 pounds a month!

Note that before accepting the Batman role, Bale dropped a significant amount of weight for his role in *The Machinist*. He lost about 64 pounds, dropping from 181 to 121 by severely under-eating and working out like a maniac. This is not a recommend method to lose weight and it can be very dangerous to your health. Bale consulted with a nutritionist to make sure he was getting enough of the proper nutrients to keep him from breaking down completely, but Bale says he still couldn't even do one push-up when he started training for *Batman—The Dark Knight*.

Since Bale's normal weight was around 181 pounds, when he started eating right his weight would've started to go back up naturally. However, if he just ate without a proper nutrition plan, he'd put on more fat than lean muscle. In order to make sure the weight gain was as much solid muscle as possible, he had to train with heavy weights to rebuild his strength and muscle mass. But he also had to make sure his diet was spot on—

just the right amount of protein from lean meats and fish, lots of fresh vegetables and some healthy fats. His starchy carb intake (potatoes, grains, breads) and his alcohol consumption would be very minimal since both grains/cereals and alcohol will fatten you up pretty fast.

In addition to weight training, Bale did a variety of bodyweight exercises, such as sprints, push-ups and pull-ups. He also did some martial arts training to improve his hand-eye coordination, hand and foot speed and overall mobility and flexibility.

Can you do it? It'd be very tough for anyone to gain 100 pounds of mostly muscle mass in six months, but you can certainly pack on 10 to 15 pounds in that time by following Bale's workout and eating right.

The Workout

Bale's routine is on the internet with some variations. It consists of 3 workouts per week and one workout that's active rest. This 12-week program will pack on some mass to your chest, back and legs. It'll also improve explosive power in both your chest and legs. On top of that, Sprint Day will really ramp up your heart rate.

Day 1 targets upper-body and back development with chin-ups, rows, high pulls and cleans. Day 2 focuses on lower-body power with sprints, squat jumps and reverse lunges. Day 3 is chest day. We've added barbell deadlifts to the routine because the glutes and hamstrings weren't being worked enough in this routine. Bale's routine is very

quadriceps dominant and even though the power cleans should be using the glutes and hamstrings (posterior chain), many people use the quads too much.

Day 4 is an active recovery day, which means do something moderate that you enjoy. In Bale's case it was swimming, but it could be tai chi, yoga, golf or anything at a light intensity that helps you relax. Bale's routine also called for him to spend 30 minutes or so stretching, although he should've been stretching 10 minutes or so after every workout to maintain his flexibility.

In addition to active recovery, you should do soft tissue work with foam rollers and similar tools to increase blood flow to the muscles, release trigger points and "unstick" muscle fibers and fascia. Many do this prior to their workout but you can do it after as well. If you have time, do both. At the end of each workout you should also be stretching out the muscles you worked to keep from getting too tight and rigid. You can have big muscles and still move well. Bale practiced martial arts on his off days, not only for the fight scene prep but also to keep his movements fast and fluid.

We highly recommend getting a good deep-tissue massage on Day 5 or 6 to complement your yoga/stretching. Recovery is important—without it, your muscles won't grow and you'll feel terrible. If you have a day where you don't feel up to the day's workout, either take the day off or do your active recovery work instead.

Weeks 1–4

Each week try to add a little more weight to the bar but don't sacrifice form to go heavier.

Monday			Back & Full-Body Power		
	Sets	Reps	Time/Tempo	Rest	Notes
1a) Chin-Ups	4	12			superset: do A followed by B, continuing until you've finished all sets of each
1b) Barbell Bent Rows	4	12	2-1-1		
3 minutes rest					
2) Barbell High Pulls		12/10/8/6		45 sec after each set	increase weight if possible as reps go down
3 minutes rest					
3) Barbell Power Cleans		12/10/8/6		90 sec after each set	increase weight if possible as reps go down
3 minutes rest					
4) Barbell Presses		10/8/6		90 sec after each set	increase weight if possible as reps go down
Tuesday			Rest: do some stretching or a light bodyweight workout.		
Wednesday			Legs		
1) Sprints	4–6		5 sec	15 sec	max effort
5 minutes rest					
2a) Squat Jumps	4	AMRAP			superset
2b) Super Plank	4	10			
3) Reverse Lunges	4	10 R/L		1 min	
Thursday			Rest: do some stretching or a light bodyweight workout.		
Friday			Chest		
1) Explosive Bench Presses	3	10	explosive	2 min	use a spotter
2) Dumbbell Flyes	3	10		2 min	
3) Clapping Push-Ups	3	AMRAP		1 min	
4) Deadlifts		12/10/8	1 min	1 min	increase weight if possible as reps go down
Saturday			Active Recovery: moderate walk, swimming, yoga, etc.		
Sunday			Rest: do some stretching or a light bodyweight workout.		

Weeks 5–8

Monday			Full Body & Back		
	Sets	*Reps*	*Time/Tempo*	*Rest*	*Notes*
1a) Pull-Ups	5	AMRAP		30 sec	superset: do A followed by B, continuing until you've finished all sets of each
1b) Dumbbell Rows	5	5 R/L		30 sec	
2 minutes rest					
2) Barbell High Pulls	5	5		2–3 min	
2 minutes rest					
3) Barbell Power Cleans	5	5		2–3 min	
2 minutes rest					
4) Barbell Presses	5	5		2–3 min	
Tuesday	Rest: do some stretching or a light bodyweight workout.				
Wednesday			Legs		
1) Sprints	4–6		5 sec	20 sec	
5 minutes rest					
2) Squat Jumps	3	10		1 min	use an external load (KB, sandbag, weight vest) ONLY if you can do at least 30 straight
1 minute rest					
3) Rear Foot Elevated Split Squats	3	8 R/L		45 sec	hold KB/DB at chest height like a goblet squat
Thursday	Rest: do some stretching or a light bodyweight workout.				
Friday			Chest		
1) Bench Presses	5	5		2 min	use a spotter
2) Dumbbell Flyes	3	5		2 min	
3) Explosive Push-Ups	3	AMRAP		1 min	
4) Deadlifts	5	5		2 min	
Saturday	Active Recovery: moderate walk, swimming, yoga, etc.				
Sunday	Rest: do some stretching or a light bodyweight workout.				

Weeks 9–12
This series returns to muscle building with a bit more metabolic conditioning.

Monday

	Sets	Reps	Time/Tempo	Rest	Notes
1a) Inverted Rows	3	15	2-1-2		superset: do A followed by B, continuing until you've finished all sets of each
1b) ½ Kneeling Band Pulls	3	10 R/L	2-1-2		
2 minutes rest					
2a) Barbell/DB/KB Shrugs	3	12			superset
2b) KB Double Dead Cleans	3	12			
2 minutes rest					
3) KB/DB Double Presses	3	8		1 min	

Tuesday
Rest: do some stretching or a light bodyweight workout.

Wednesday — Sprints/Legs

	Sets	Reps	Time/Tempo	Rest	Notes
1a) Sprints	4–6		5 sec	15 sec	superset
1b) 2-Hand KB Swings	4–6	20		15 sec	
2 minutes rest					
2a) Jump Squats	3	10			superset • for squats elevate and hold a DB/KB between your legs, arms extended • for lunges alternate legs for 20 TOTAL reps
2b) Reverse Lunge to Forward Lunges	3	20			

Thursday
Rest: do some stretching or a light bodyweight workout.

Friday

	Sets	Reps	Time/Tempo	Rest	Notes
1) DB/KB Floor Presses	5	10 R/L	2-1-2		
2 minutes rest					
2) Dips	3	AMRAP		30 sec	
3) Quad Hops	3	AMRAP		30 sec	
4) Deadlifts	5	10		1 min	

Saturday
Active Recovery: moderate walk, swimming, yoga, etc.

Sunday
Rest: do some stretching or a light bodyweight workout.

JESSICA BIEL
WORKOUT APPROACH FOR
ABIGAIL WHISTLER—BLADE 3: TRINITY

With her lean, firm muscles and defined shoulders, arms, butt and back, Jessica Biel looked like the strong, tough vampire hunter she was in *Blade 3: Trinity*, the film in which she co-starred with Wesley Snipes. She lost about 10 pounds of fat training for *Blade 3* but she also packed on several pounds of very good-looking muscle.

Biel is 5'7" and her weight has ranged from 105 to 117 pounds. As a child she was a gymnast and played soccer. Some websites say she had 6–8% body fat for this movie, but we doubt it. Women who are that lean face all sorts of hormonal imbalances and she would've had a very drawn-in face and no curves. Her weight was probably closer to the high end during *Blade 3* and her body fat was more like 16–18%, which is considered to be as lean as a woman can be and still remain healthy.

The fact that her weight fluctuated and that she was probably closer to 117 pounds during *Blade 3* goes to show why women shouldn't get concerned about what the scale says. Instead, focus on what you look like without clothes on and whether you find yourself needing to buy smaller outfits.

Biel's latest role is in the remake of *Total Recall*, in which she plays Melina who helps Quaid (the role originally played by Arnold Schwarzenegger) fight the bad guys and save the world. In this role she appears to have lost some of her muscularity but still looks like she can kick serious butt.

The Workout

Six weeks before shooting began, Biel and the other *Blade 3* actors trained for 4 hours almost every day. Her 6-days-per-week program lasted 2 months and consisted of conditioning and weight training, sprinting for various distances, plyometrics (jumping), lunge variations for her butt, rows for her upper back and shoulders, curls for her biceps, and Russian twists and hanging leg raises for the core. Essentially, Biel spent 45 minutes on cardio (for fat loss), 1 hour on strength training (to build muscle and burn more fat), 1 hour on martial arts training and another hour on archery practice. She said archery was the hardest because of the precision required to shoot accurately.

In Biel's original workout her trainer had her sprint for 200 meters, which is pretty demanding. Even if top sprinters run 100 meters in about 10 seconds, going 200 meters is a long distance for the average person. You can't maintain maximum output for that long, so sprint for 3 to 5 seconds; as you get better you can increase that to 5 to 8 seconds and eventually up to 10 seconds. Then work on doing it 2 or 3 times.

Her trainer also had her jumping up flights of stairs 3 at a time. While that's a great way to build muscle and strength in the lower body, especially the butt, it's also a very advanced movement and if you miss, you get to kiss the steps. For beginners we prefer step-ups progressing to low box jumps (half shin height) and working up from there.

Of course, no one with a life has 4 hours to train and you can only sustain that level of intensity for a short period of time before getting injured or having your body break down. Rest is a big factor in your training and without adequate rest you may never fulfill your goals.

The following program is what we've designed to safely and effectively help you mold yourself in the likeness of Jessica Biel. It's a 4-week program designed to be done either Monday/Wednesday/Friday or Tuesday/Thursday/Saturday. You can extend this workout for up to 12 weeks. There's enough variety but still enough sameness that you won't get bored and your body will continue to positively adapt to the training. If you do take it to 8 or 12 weeks, you should be able to use heavier weights each successive cycle.

Week 1

Monday	Sets	Reps	Time/Tempo	Rest	Notes
1) Jog	1		5 min	1 min	
2) Sprint	3		3–5 sec	30 sec walk/ jog	as these get easier over time, take shorter rests down to about 15 sec then go longer and increase the rest again
			2 minutes rest		
3a) BB/KB Romanian Deadlifts	4	8	3-1-2		tri-set: do A followed by B and C, continuing until you've finished all sets of each
3b) Dumbbell Curls	4	8 R/L	2-1-3		
3c) DB/KB Triceps Extensions	4	8			
				2 min	
4a) ½ Kneeling Band Pulls	4	10 R/L	3-1-3		superset
4b) 1-Hand KB Swings	4	15 R/L			
			2 minutes rest		
5a) Walkouts/Ab Rollouts	3	10			tri-set
5b) Split Squats: L1–No Weight L2–Goblet L3–Rack (same side as back leg) L4–Overhead (same side as back leg)	3	10 R/L			
5c) Unicycles	3	20 R/L			
			1 minute rest		
6a) Squat Thrusts	8 (4 min)		L1–10 L2–15 L3–20	20 sec 15 sec 10 sec	superset • depending on your conditioning level do the squat thrust for the time specified, rest the appropriate interval then do the push-ups using the same work-to-rest interval for a total of 8 times or 4 min
6b) Push-Ups			L1–10 L2–15 L3–20	20 sec 15 sec 10 sec	

Tuesday	Rest: do some stretching or a light bodyweight workout.				
Wednesday	*Sets*	*Reps*	*Time/Tempo*	*Rest*	*Notes*
1) Jump Rope	1		5 min	1 min	
2) L1–Step-Ups L2–Weighted Step-Ups L3–Low Box Jumps L4–Knee-High Box Jumps L5–Mid-Thigh Box Jumps	1	L1-L2–8 R/L L3-L5–20			for L2 hold 1 KB goblet style
		2 minutes rest			
3a) Squats (Barbell Front Squat or KB/DB Goblet Squat)	4	8		1 min	superset: do A followed by B, continuing until you've finished all sets of each
3b) L1–Split Squats L2–Front Lunges L3–Reverse Lunges L4–Walking Lunges L5–Jumping Lunges	4	L1–8 R/L L2-L5–8 R/L alternating legs		1 min	
		2 minutes rest			
4a) DB/KB Overhead Presses	4	10 R/L	2-1-2		superset
4b) Low Windmills	4	10 R/L	2-1-2		
		2 minutes rest			
5a) L1–Dead Bug L2–Leg Thrusts L3–Hanging Knee Raises L4–Hanging Leg Raises	3	L1–20 total L2-L4–10		30 sec	superset
5b) L1–Side Plank L2–Rotational Side Plank L3–Side Plank w/ Hip Lift	3	15 R/L		1 min	
6a) 2-Hand Swings	3		30 sec	30 sec	tri-set
6b) Super Plank	3		30 sec	30 sec	
6c) Squat Thrusts	3		30 sec	1 min	

Thursday		Rest: do some stretching or a light bodyweight workout.				
Friday	*Sets*	*Reps*	*Time/Tempo*	*Rest*	*Notes*	
1a) 2-Hand Swings	1		30 sec		tri-set: do A followed by B and C, continuing until you've finished all sets of each	
1b) 1-Hand Swings	1		30 sec R, 30 sec L			
1c) H2H Swings	1		30 sec			
1 minute rest						
2) Barbell High Pulls	1	10				
1 minute rest						
3a) KB 1-Hand High Pulls	4	10 R/L			superset	
3b) KB/DB Rows	4	10 R/L				
2 minutes rest						
4a) Inverted Rows	4	10	3-1-2		superset	
4b) Weighted Glute Bridges	4	10	1-5-1		• for glute bridges use a KB/DB just below navel or use a band across hips	
2 minutes rest						
5a) Plank & Reach	4	15			superset	
5b) Pullover Crunches	4	12		30 sec		
1 minute rest						
6a) Figure 8s w/ Hold	3		30 sec	15 sec	circuit	
6b) Slingshots	3		30 sec R/L	15 sec after 2nd side		
6c) KB Swing Flip & Squat	3		30 sec	15 sec		
6d) Jumping Jacks	3		30 sec	1 min		
Saturday		Rest: do some stretching or a light bodyweight workout.				
Sunday		Rest: do some stretching or a light bodyweight workout.				

Week 2

Monday	Sets	Reps	Time /Tempo	Rest	Notes
1) Light Jog	1		5 min	1 min	
2) Sprint	3		3–5 sec	jog/walk 30 sec	
2 minutes rest					
3a) 1-Leg Romanian Deadlifts	4	8 R/L	312		superset: do A followed by B, continuing until you've finished all sets of each
3b) Barbell Curls	4	8–10			
1 minute rest					
4a) Inverted Rows	4	10 R/L			superset
4b) Floor Presses	4	10 R/L			
1 minute rest					
5a) Walkouts/Ab Rollouts	4	10			tri-set
5b) Weighted Glute Bridges	4	10			
5c) Low or High Windmills	4	8 R/L			
1 minute rest					
6a) Mountain Climbers	4		20	10 sec	
6b) Jumping Jacks	4		20	10 sec	
6c) Squat Thrusts	4		20	10 sec	
30–60 seconds rest after each tri-set					
Tuesday	Rest: do some stretching or a light bodyweight workout.				

Wednesday	Sets	Reps	Time/Tempo	Rest	Notes
1) Jump Rope	1		5 min	1 min	

2) L1—Step-Ups
   L2—Low Box Jumps
   L3—Knee-High Box Jumps
   L4—Mid-Thigh Box Jumps
	3	L1—8 R/L
		L2-L4—20
				30 sec	

1 minute rest					
3a) Goblet Squats	3	10	2-1-2		tri-set: do A followed by B and C, continuing until you've finished all sets of each

3b) Bird Dogs:
   L1—1 Arm
   L2—1 Leg
   L3—1 Arm & Opposite Leg
	3	10 R/L	1-4-1		

3c) Rear Foot Elevated Split Squats	3	10 R/L	2-0-2		
1 minute rest					
4a) KB/DB Tall Kneeling Overhead Presses	3	8 R/L			superset
4b) 2-Hand KB/DB Chest Presses	3	10			
1 minute rest					

5a) L1—Dead Bug
   L2—Leg Thrusts
   L3—Hanging Knee Raises
   L4—Hanging Leg Raises
	3	AMRAP		30 sec	superset

5b) Super Plank	3	10		30 sec	
6a) KB Dead Cleans			30 sec R/L	15 sec	circuit: repeat up to 3x if possible
6b) Jumping Jacks			30 sec	15 sec	
6c) Mountain Climbers			30 sec	15 sec	
6d) Split Squats			30 sec R/L	1 min	
Thursday	Rest: do some stretching or a light bodyweight workout.				

Friday	Sets	Reps	Time/Tempo	Rest	Notes
1a) 2-Hand KB Swings	1		30 sec		tri-set: do A followed by B and C, continuing until you've finished all sets of each
1b) 1-Hand Swings	1		30 sec R, 30 sec L		
1c) H2H Swings	1		30 sec		
1 minute rest					
2) Barbell High Pulls	3	8		1 min	go heavy
1 minute rest					
3a) Dead Cleans	3	12 R/L		15–30 sec	superset
3b) Lunge to Step-Ups	3	15 R/L		15–30 sec	
1 minute rest					
4a) KB/DB Rows	3	12 R/L		15–30 sec	superset
4b) ½ Kneeling Band Pulls	3	10 R/L		15–30 sec	
1 minute rest					
5a) Farmer's Walk	3		60 sec	30 sec	superset • go heavy, use 2 bells
5b) Waiter's Walk	3		30 sec R/L	30 sec	heavy as possible but keep elbow straight
1 minute rest					
6a) 1-Hand KB High Pulls			30 sec R/L	15 sec	superset: repeat up to 3x
6b) Mountain Climbers			30 sec	15 sec	
Saturday	Rest: do some stretching or a light bodyweight workout.				
Sunday	Rest: do some stretching or a light bodyweight workout.				

Week 3

Monday	Sets	Reps	Time/Tempo	Rest	Notes
1) Jog	1		5 min	1 min	
2) Sprint	4		3–5 sec	20 sec	
2 minutes rest					
1a) Pull-Ups	4	AMRAP			superset: do A followed by B, continuing until you've finished all sets of each
1b) Barbell/KB Romanian Deadlifts	4	5			
2 minutes rest					
2a) KB/DB Floor Presses	4	5 R/L			superset
2b) DB/KB Rows	4	5			
2 minutes rest					
3a) Step-Ups	4	5 R/L			superset
3b) Side Lunges	4	5 R/L			
1 minute rest					
4a) Forearm Plank	1		2 min	30 sec	superset
4b) Side Plank	1		90 sec R/L		
1 minute rest					
5a) KB Dead Cleans	4		30 sec R/L	15 sec	circuit
5b) Slingshots	4		30 sec R	15 sec	
5c) Figure 8s w/ Hold	4		30 sec	15 sec	
5d) Slingshots	4		30 sec L	30 sec	
Tuesday	Rest: do some stretching or a light bodyweight workout.				

Wednesday	Sets	Reps	Time/Tempo	Rest	Notes
1) Jump Rope	1		3–5 min	2 min	
2) L1—Step-Ups 　　L2—Low Box Jumps 　　L3—Knee-High Box Jumps 　　L4—Mid-Thigh Box Jumps	1	L1-8 R/L L2-L4—20			
3a) Squats (Barbell Front Squat 　　or KB/DB Goblet Squat)	4	5	2-0-2		superset: do A followed by B, continuing until you've finished all sets of each
3b) Push-Ups	4	AMRAP	2-1-1		
2 minutes rest					
4a) Dumbbell Curls	4	5 R/L	1-1-3		superset
4b) KB/DB Triceps Extensions	4	5	1-1-1		
1 minute rest					
5a) Lunge variations	4	8 R/L			superset
5b) Low Windmills	4	5 R/L			
6a) 2-Hand KB Swings	1	20			tri-set • use the same bell for all the swings in this circuit; try to complete without stopping
6b) 1-Hand KB Swings	1	20 R/L			
6c) H2H KB Swings	1	20			
7) Farmer's Walk	4 laps		100 ft		switch hands each lap; the KB/DB should be heavy enough for you to feel it but not so much you can't maintain posture
Thursday	Rest: do some stretching or a light bodyweight workout.				

Friday	Sets	Reps	Time/Tempo	Rest	Notes
1) Light Jog	1		5 min	1 min	
2) Sprint	4		5 sec	20 sec	
2 minutes rest					
3a) 2-Hand KB Swings	5	20			circuit
3b) KB/DB Overhead Presses	5	5 R/L			
3c) KB/DB Goblet Squats	5	5			
3d) 2-Hand KB/DB Chest Presses	5	5			
2 minutes rest					
4a) Kettlebell Dead Cleans	5	5			tri-set
4b) Inverted Rows	5	8			
4c) Walkouts/Ab Rollouts	5	10			
2 minutes rest					
5) Offset Walk	6 laps		50 ft/lap		1 light bell overhead, 1 heavy bell hanging down; switch each lap

HIIT	Level I	Level II	Level III	Level IV	Work/Rest
Jumping Jacks	Jumping Jacks	Jumping Jacks	Jumping Jacks	Jumping Jacks	30 sec/15 sec
Burpees	Hands Elevated	Squat Thrust (no push-up)	Burpee Level II	Full Burpee	30 sec/15 sec
Plank	High Plank	Forearm Plank	Super Plank	Super Plank	30 sec/15 sec
Side Lunges	Alternating Side Lunge	Alternating Step-out Side Lunge	Skater's Lunge	Skater's Lunge	30 sec/15 sec

Week 4

Monday	Sets	Reps	Time/Tempo	Rest	Notes
1a) Jumping Jacks	1	50			circuit
1b) Skip	1	30 yards			
1c) Shuffle	1	30 yards			
1d) Carioca	1	30 yards			
2) Mountain Climbers	4		20	10 sec	this is a 2-min round
3 minutes rest					
3a) Barbell Romanian Deadlifts	3	10			superset: do A followed by B, continuing until you've finished all sets of each
3b) 1-Arm Standing Band Rows	3	20 R/L	1-1-1		
2 minutes rest					
4a) Stability Ball or Suspension Jack Knives	3	10			superset
4b) Dumbbell Curls	3	15 R/L			
2 minutes rest					
5a) Rear Foot Elevated Split Squats	3	10 R/L			superset
5b) Horizontal Band Chest Pull-Aparts	3	10			
2 minutes rest					
6) 1-Hand KB High Pulls		10/12/14/ 16/18/20/ 10 R/L		time it takes to do the reps	

Tuesday	Rest: do some stretching or a light bodyweight workout.				
Wednesday	*Sets*	*Reps*	*Time/Tempo*	*Rest*	*Notes*
Jump Rope	1		5 min	1 min	

2) L1–Step-Ups
  L2–Low Box Jumps
  L3–Knee-High Box Jumps
  L4–Mid-Thigh Box Jumps
	2	L1–8 R/L
		L2–L4 20
				30 sec	

		2 minutes rest			
3a) Barbell Back Squats	3	8			tri-set: do A followed by B and C, continuing until you've finished all sets of each
3b) KB/DB Overhead Presses	3	10 R/L			
3c) Plank & Reach	3	20			
		2 minutes rest			
4a) Step-Ups	3	12 R/L			tri-set
4b) KB/DB Floor Presses	3	12 R/L			
4c) Unicycles	3	20 R/L			
		2 minutes rest			
5a) Ropes: Double Waves	8		15 sec	15 sec	circuit
5b) Ropes: Alternating Waves	8		15 sec	15 sec	
5c) Ropes: In/Outs	8		15 sec	15 sec	
5d) Ropes: Alternating Slams	8		15 sec	30 sec	
Thursday	Rest: do some stretching or a light bodyweight workout.				

Friday	Sets	Reps	Time/Tempo	Rest	Notes
1) Light Jog	1		5 min	1 min	
2a) Sprint	1		10 sec	30 sec	tri-set: do A followed by B and C, continuing until you've finished all sets of each
2b) Sprint	1		8 sec	20 sec	
2c) Sprint	1		5 sec		
1 minute rest					
3a) 2-Hand KB Swings	4	20			superset
3b) Diagonal Band Chest Pull-Aparts	4	10 R/L	212		• for pull-aparts alternate each rep
1 minute rest					
4a) Pull-Ups	3	AMRAP			superset
4b) Stability Ball or Suspension Trainer Hamstring Curls	3	12			
2 minutes rest					

5a) Lunges
  L1–Static Lunges
  L2–Forward Lunges
  L3–Reverse Lunges
  L4–Walking Lunges
  L5–Jumping Lunges
	4	L1–8 R/L
		L2-L5–8 R/L alternating legs
					superset

5b) Push-Ups	4	AMRAP at least 10			
1 minute rest					
6a) 2-Hand KB Swings	8		15 sec		circuit
6b) Mountain Climbers	8		15 sec		
6c) Jumping Jacks	8		15 sec		
6d) Squats	8		15 sec		
Saturday	Rest: do some stretching or a light bodyweight workout.				
Sunday	Rest: do some stretching or a light bodyweight workout.				

HENRY CAVILL
WORKOUT APPROACH FOR
SUPERMAN—MAN OF STEEL

British actor Henry Cavill was called the "fat kid" when he was growing up and was rather soft even during his time as Charles Brandon in the Showtime series *The Tudors*. When he was chosen for the role of Theseus in *The Immortals*, the director told him he needed to shape up and get an eight pack. With hard work, he was able to achieve an extremely lean, wiry and athletic look with around 6% body fat.

While working on *The Immortals*, Cavill was cast in *Man of Steel* as Clark Kent/Superman. As soon as filming for *The Immortals* was done, he had to switch gears to bulk up for his new role. Cavill ate around 3000 calories per day during filming for *The Immortals*. When he started training for Superman, he had to up that amount to around 5000 calories per day.

THE WORKOUT

According to Cavill, he spent an hour or 2 training every morning for his *Immortals* role before filming *The Tudors*, and again after filming was done for the day. Once shooting for *The Tudors* finished and he started work on *The Immortals*, his workouts were shorter (mostly high-intensity interval training using bodyweight) but just as tough because they included sword fighting and martial arts in addition to his usual regimen.

For his role as the *Man of Steel*, Cavill needed to build some super muscle quickly. Once he wrapped up his *Immortals* work he began to build his body of steel by shifting to a bodybuilding-style workout: lifting moderate to heavy weights with reps typically in the 10 to 12 range, and many times going to failure.

In order to stay lean while adding muscle he continued to incorporate conditioning work. He was on a 5000-calorie, mostly protein diet and the high-intensity interval training he did (see workout) helped keep the fat off while the bodybuilding workouts packed on slabs of muscle—20 pounds of it!

THESEUS

The following workout is one Cavill supposedly did every day to get his body fat low for *The Immortals*. While it's a good conditioning circuit, doing this daily for months will actually cause your fat loss to slow down as the body adapts to the workout. The other issue is increased risk of injury from overuse and lack of rest/recovery. In order for the body to get stronger, burn fat or build muscle, you must have downtime— that's when the body actually undergoes changes caused by the training (or lack thereof).

Here's the circuit from *Men's Health* UK edition. It's done with little to no rest between exercises. After completing the circuit take 8 deep, controlled breaths and repeat for a total of 5 sets of the circuit, as quickly as possible. Hindu squats can be tough on the knees so substitute them with regular bodyweight squats if you need to. When

Some say Cavill did the *300* workout made famous by Gerard Butler and the cast of the movie *300* (see my other book *Spartan Warrior Workout* for details on that workout and how to train for it) because he was also trained by Mark Twight, trainer of the *300* cast and crew.

doing the bicycles, one rep is right elbow/left knee and then left elbow/right knee.

If you're new to high-intensity interval training (HIIT), take your time and build up to it. For beginners, rest between each exercise until your heart rate drops to about 120–130 beats per minute. I wouldn't do this workout more than 3 days per week (say Monday/ Wednesday/Friday). On the other days, depending on your goals, do either strength training or use a more bodybuilding approach, as we'll talk about below. Make sure you incorporate rest days as well—it's the most important part of your workout!

25 Hindu Push-Ups

25 Hindu Squats

25 Bicycles

25 Squat Thrusts

Besides doing this for reps, try using a timer and doing intervals of 20 seconds of work, 10 seconds of rest, and then moving to the next exercise. Repeat the circuit 5 times. If that's easy, do 30/15 intervals instead of 20/10, or add a weight vest. Take minimal rest between circuits.

SUPERMAN

This 4-week, 3-days-per-week routine can help you become a superman. While you won't be able to fly, you'll feel ready to leap tall buildings in a single bound. The first and third weeks focus on volume, lifting moderately heavy weights for 3 sets of 8–12 reps. This is considered the typical bodybuilder bulking program. During weeks two and four you'll focus on building strength, working with heavier weights in a 5-sets-of-5 setup, the typical "strength" program.

After doing this 4-week program you'll look and feel like you can stop a bullet (but don't try it) and you won't have to worry about kryptonite sapping your super powers.

Week 1

Monday	Sets	Reps	Time/Tempo	Rest	Notes
1a) Bench Presses	3	8	3-1-2		superset: do A followed by B, continuing until you've finished all sets of each
1b) Barbell Bent Rows	3	8	3-1-2		
			2 minutes rest		
2a) Incline Bench Presses	3	10	3-1-2		superset
2b) Pull-Ups	3	AMRAP			
			2 minutes rest		
3a) 1-Arm Bench or Floor Presses	3	10 R/L	2-1-3		superset
3b) Heavy-Resistance Band or Cable Pulls	3	10 R/L	2-1-3		• for floor presses explode up, pause, slow descent • for pulls explode on the pull, hold, then slowly return. No cheating!
			2 minutes rest		
4a) Dumbbell Flyes	3	10			superset
4b) Reverse Flyes	3	10			

Tuesday	Rest: do some stretching or a light bodyweight workout.				
Wednesday	*Sets*	*Reps*	*Time/Tempo*	*Rest*	*Notes*
1a) Barbell Front Squats	3	8	3-0-2		superset: do A followed by B, continuing until you've finished all sets of each
1b) Super Plank	3	AMRAP			
		2 minutes rest			
2a) Lunge variations	3	10 R/L			superset
2b) Unicycles	3	25 R/L			
		2 minutes rest			
3a) Barbell Deadlifts	3	8	2-1-2		superset
3b) Low Windmills	3	6	2-1-2		
		2 minutes rest			
4a) Ab Rollouts	3	AMRAP			superset
4b) Calf Raises	3	8–10			
		2 minutes rest			
5a) Barbell Good Mornings	3	10			superset
5b) Weighted Glute Bridges	3	10	2-2-2		
Thursday	Rest: do some stretching or a light bodyweight workout.				
Friday	*Sets*	*Reps*	*Time/Tempo*	*Rest*	*Notes*
1a) Barbell Curls	3	10	1-1-2		superset
1b) KB/DB Triple Crush	3	10			
		2 minutes rest			
2a) Barbell Overhead Presses	3	8			superset
2b) DB/KB Shrugs	3	10	1-2-1		
		2 minutes rest			
3a) Dips	3	AMRAP			superset
3b) Kettlebell Push-Ups	3	AMRAP			
		2 minutes rest			

	Sets	Reps	Time/Tempo	Rest	Notes
4a) Dumbbell Hammer Curls	3	10 R/L	1-1-2		superset: do A followed by B, continuing until you've finished all sets of each
4b) Barbell Reverse Curls	3	10 R/L			
2 minutes rest					
5a) Farmer's Walk	3		60 sec	30 sec	superset
5b) Heavy-Resistance Band 1-Arm Triceps Extensions	3	8			
Saturday	Rest: do some stretching or a light bodyweight workout.				
Sunday	Rest: do some stretching or a light bodyweight workout.				

Week 2

This is the same as Week 1, just with more sets and fewer reps. Go heavier!

Monday	*Sets*	*Reps*	*Time/Tempo*	*Rest*	*Notes*
1a) Bench Presses	5	5			superset
1b) Barbell Bent Rows	5	5			
2 minutes rest					
2a) Incline Bench Presses	5	5			superset
2b) Pull-Ups	5	AMRAP			
2 minutes rest					
3a) 1-Arm Bench or Floor Presses	5	6 R/L			superset
3b) Heavy-Resistance Band or Cable Pulls	5	6 R/L			
2 minutes rest					
4a) Dumbbell Flyes	5	5			superset
4b) Reverse Flyes	5	5			

Wednesday (week 2)	Sets	Reps	Time/Tempo	Rest	Notes
1a) Barbell Front Squats	5	5			superset: do A followed by B, continuing until you've finished all sets of each
1b) Super Plank	5	AMRAP			
2 minutes rest					
2a) Lunge variations	5	5 R/L			superset
2b) Unicycles	5	5 R/L			
2 minutes rest					
3a) Barbell Deadlifts	5	5	2-1-2		superset
3b) Low Windmills	5	5	2-1-2		
2 minutes rest					
4a) Ab Rollouts	5	AMRAP			superset
4b) Calf Raises	5	8–10			
2 minutes rest					
5a) Barbell Good Mornings	5	5			superset
5b) Weighted Glute Bridges	5	5			
Thursday	Rest: do some stretching or a light bodyweight workout.				
Friday					
1a) Barbell Curls	5	5	1-1-2		superset
1b) KB/DB Triple Crushes	5	5			
2 minutes rest					
2a) Barbell Overhead Presses	5	5			superset
2b) DB/KB Shrugs	5	5	1-2-1		
2 minutes rest					
3a) Dips	5	AMRAP			superset
3b) Kettlebell Push-Ups	5	AMRAP			
2 minutes rest					
4a) Dumbbell Hammer Curls	5	5 R/L			superset
4b) Barbell Reverse Curls	5	5 R/L			

		2 minutes rest			
5a) Farmer's Walk	5		60	30 sec	superset: do A followed by B, continuing until you've finished all sets of each
5b) Heavy-Resistance Band 1-Arm Triceps Extensions	5	5			

Week 3

Monday	Sets	Reps	Time/Tempo	Rest	Notes
1a) Double KB Floor Presses	3	8	3-1-2		superset
1b) DB/KB Bent Rows	3	8	3-1-2		
		2 minutes rest			
2a) Decline Bench Presses	3	10	3-1-2		superset
2b) Pull-Ups	3	AMRAP			
		2 minutes rest			
3a) ½ Kneeling Band Chest Presses	3	10 R/L	3-1-2		superset • if rows are easy, use a weight vest
3b) Inverted Rows	3	10	2-1-3		
		2 minutes rest			
4a) Suspended Face-Down Flyes	3	10			superset
4b) Suspended Face-Up Flyes	3	10			
Tuesday	Rest; do some stretching or a light bodyweight workout.				
Wednesday					
1a) Back Squats	3	8	3-0-2		superset
1b) Leg Thrusts	3	AMRAP			
		2 minutes rest			
2a) Rear Foot Elevated Split Squats	3	10 R/L			superset • do split squats with bar on shoulders, KB/DB in front or 1-arm hanging
2b) Rotational Band Pulls	3	10 R/L			
		2 minutes rest			
3a) KB/DB Sumo Deadlifts	3	8			superset
3b) Side Plank w/ Hip Raise (weighted)	3	15 R/L			

Wednesday (continued, week 2)

		2 minutes rest			
4a) Ab Rollouts	3	AMRAP			superset: do A followed by B, continuing until you've finished all sets of each
4b) Calf Raises	3	15			
		1 minute rest			
5a) Back Extensions	3	10		30 sec	superset ▪ for back extensions use a stability ball if you don't have an extension apparatus
5b) Stability Ball Hamstring Curls	5	10 R/L		30 sec	

Thursday — Rest: do some stretching or a light bodyweight workout.

Friday	Sets	Reps	Time/Tempo	Rest	Notes
1a) EZ-Bar Curls	3	10	1-1-2		superset
1b) Skull Crushers	3	10			
		2 minutes rest			
2a) Double KB/DB Presses	3	10			superset ▪ go heavy!
2b) KB/DB Suitcase Deadlifts	3	10			
		2 minutes rest			
3a) Barbell Forearm Curls	3	AMRAP			superset
3b) Wrist Rollers	3	AMRAP			
		2 minutes rest			
4a) 1-Arm Heavy-Resistance Band Curls	3	10 R/L			superset
4b) Dumbbell Kickbacks	3	10 R/L			
		2 minutes rest			
5a) Offset Walk	3		60	30 sec	superset
5b) 2-Arm Heavy-Resistance Band Bent-Over Triceps Extensions	3	10			

Week 4

Monday	Sets	Reps	Time/Tempo	Rest	Notes
1a) Double KB Floor Presses	5	5	3-1-2		superset: do A followed by B, continuing until you've finished all sets of each
1b) DB/KB Bent Rows	5	5	3-1-2		
2 minutes rest					
2a) Decline Bench Presses	5	5	3-1-2		superset
2b) Pull-Ups	5	AMRAP			
2 minutes rest					
3a) ½ Kneeling Band Chest Presses	5	5 R/L	3-1-2		superset • if rows are easy use a weight vest
3b) Inverted Rows	5	5	2-1-3		
2 minutes rest					
4a) Suspended Face-Down Flyes	5	5			superset
4b) Suspended Face-Up Flyes	5	5			
Tuesday	Rest: do some stretching or a light bodyweight workout.				
Wednesday					
1a) Back Squats	3	8	3-0-2		superset
1b) Leg Thrusts	3	AMRAP			
2 minutes rest					
2a) Rear Foot Elevated Split Squats	3	10 R/L			superset • do split squats with bar on shoulders, KB/DB in front or 1-arm hanging • band pulls are explosive
2b) Rotational Band Pulls	3	10 R/L			
2 minutes rest					
3a) KB/DB Sumo Deadlifts	3	8			superset
3b) Side Plank w/ Hip Raise (weighted)	3	15 R/L			
2 minutes rest					

Wednesday (continued, week 4)

4a) Ab Rollouts	5	AMRAP			superset: do A followed by B, continuing until you've finished all sets of each
4b) Calf Raises	5	15			
		2 minutes rest			
5a) Back Extensions	5	5			superset
5b) Stability Ball Hamstring Curls	5	10 R/L			• for back extensions use a stability ball if you don't have an extension apparatus

Thursday	Rest: do some stretching or a light bodyweight workout.

Friday	Sets	Reps	Time/Tempo	Rest	Notes
1a) EZ-Bar Curls	5	5	1-1-2		superset
1b) Skull Crushers	5	5			
		2 minutes rest			
2a) Double KB/DB Presses	5	5			superset
2b) Suitcase Deadlifts	5	10			
		2 minutes rest			
3a) Barbell Forearm Curls	5	AMRAP			superset
3b) Wrist Rollers	5	AMRAP			
		2 minutes rest			
4a) 1-Arm Heavy-Resistance Band Curls	5	5 R/L			superset
4b) Dumbbell Kickbacks	5	5 R/L			
		2 minutes rest			
5a) Farmer's Walk	5		60	30 sec	superset
5b) 1-Arm Heavy-Resistance Band Triceps Extensions	5	5			

Saturday	Rest: do some stretching or a light bodyweight workout.
Sunday	Rest: do some stretching or a light bodyweight workout.

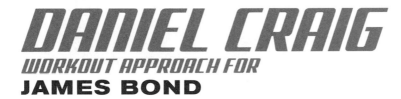

DANIEL CRAIG
WORKOUT APPROACH FOR
JAMES BOND

Unlike all of the previous actors who portrayed the super-cool British spy James Bond, athletic Daniel Craig did many of the stunts and fight scenes in *Casino Royale*, *Quantum of Solace* and *Skyfall*, his three 007 films. The focus in the 1960s wasn't on six-pack abs, just being trim and athletic looking, so there wasn't much demand to "get in shape." Sean Connery looked good but the fight choreography wasn't nearly as sophisticated as it is today. The same holds true for Roger Moore, who probably was the least athletic and in shape of the Bond actors.

Craig got strong and put on some serious muscle. According to various internet sources, Craig is anywhere from 5'10" to 6' but nowhere does it give his weight before or after his first Bond role in *Casino Royale*. Looking at some of his pictures he was probably about 175–180 pounds and 8–10% body fat. His workouts made his chest big, probably a little bigger than one would expect from someone who swims a lot (Bond is a swimmer in the books by Ian Fleming); swimmers are typically lean, strong and agile, not bulky.

The Workout

This is the workout Craig did to get his Bond body into great shape. Between the weight lifting, bodyweight exercises and martial arts work, Craig became an all-around athlete who was able to do his own stunts and fight scenes and make them look authentic. There are many similarities between the workouts done by Craig, Hugh Jackman (page 61) and Christian Bale (page 20). Since they were all trying to get bigger through the chest and back, they did similar exercises with similar sets and reps. With Craig's workout, just as with the others, you should strive for excellent form while trying to go up in weight each week.

This workout is decent but, for a power workout as done on Monday and Friday, consider splitting the clean and press into its parts and doing 3 sets of 6–8 power cleans and 3 sets of 8–10 presses. This allows you to work heavier on the true "power" portion

and still work with the correct weight on the press. In a compound movement you're limited by the weakest link in it, in this case the press.

After 4 to 6 weeks, you need to switch things up by either changing to a completely different workout or modifying this one. What you do depends on your goals. To get stronger, modify this one by dropping the reps to the 4–6 range and increasing the sets from 4 to 5. Dropping the reps allows you to use heavier weights while maintaining proper form. Adding additional sets means you'll still be moving a lot of weight over time. This will make you very strong. Continue to keep the rest periods short and you'll get plenty of "cardio" while you develop your strength. With the bodyweight exercises (pull-ups, chin-ups and dips), either increase the reps or add weight by wearing a weight vest.

Monday — Power Circuit

	Sets	Reps	Time/Tempo	Rest	Notes
1a) Clean & Press	3	10		minimal rest between exercises	superset: do A followed by B, continuing until you've finished all sets of each
Option—1a) Power Cleans	3	6–8			
Option—1b) Press	3	10			
1b) Weighted Knee Raises	3	10			
2 minutes rest					
2a) Weighted Step-Ups	3	10 R/L		minimal rest between exercises	superset
2b) Chin-Ups	3	10			
2 minutes rest					
3a) Decline Push-Ups	3	10		minimal rest between exercises	superset
3b) Dips	3	10			

Tuesday — Chest & Back

The original workout used chin-ups but we changed them to pull-ups to work more of the back and lats (the chin-up is more of a biceps exercise). We've also added in some barbell bent rows to work the back more.

	Sets	Reps	Time/Tempo	Rest	Notes
1a) Incline Bench Presses	4	10		minimal rest between exercises	tri-set
1b) Pull-Ups (palms out)	4	10			
1c) Barbell Bent Rows	4	10			
2 minutes rest					
2a) Decline Push-Ups	4	10		minimal rest between exercises	superset
2b) Incline DB Flyes	4	10			

Wednesday				Legs	
	Sets	Reps	Time/Tempo	Rest	Notes
1a) Barbell Back Squats	4	10		minimal rest between exercises	superset: do A followed by B, continuing until you've finished all sets of each
1b) Romanian Deadlifts	4	10			
2 minutes rest					
2a) Hamstring Curls on machine or ball	4	10		minimal rest between exercises	superset
2b) Alternating Forward Lunges	4	10			
Thursday				**Shoulders & Arms**	
1a) Incline DB Curls	4	10		minimal rest between exercises	superset
1b) Dips	4	10			
2 minutes rest					
2a) Lateral Raises	4	10		minimal rest between exercises	superset
2b) Shoulder Presses	4	10			

Friday			Power Circuit		
	Sets	Reps	Time/Tempo	Rest	Notes
1a) Clean & Press	3	10		minimal rest between exercises	superset: do A followed by B, continuing until you've finished all sets of each
Option—1a) Power Cleans	3	6–8			
Option—1b) Press	3	10			
1b) Weighted Knee Raises	3	10			
		2 minutes rest			
2a) Weighted Step-Ups	3	10 R/L		minimal rest between exercises	superset
2b) Chin-Ups	3	10			
		2 minutes rest			
3a) Decline Push-Ups	3	10		Minimal rest between exercises	superset
3b) Dips	3	10			
Saturday		Active Recovery: moderate walk, swimming, yoga, etc.			
Sunday		Stretching/Yoga			

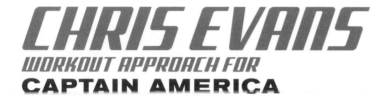

CHRIS EVANS
WORKOUT APPROACH FOR
CAPTAIN AMERICA

When Chris Evans played the Human Torch in the *Fantastic Four*, he was already in fantastic shape. At 6' tall and 160 pounds, he was pretty lean and thus needed to put on some muscle mass for his starring role in *Captain America*. Through his trainer Simon Waterson, who trained Daniel Craig for both of his Bond films, Evans gained about 20 pounds of muscle.

He went from a trim but soft build (around 160 pounds) as the Human Torch to about 180 pounds and 8–10% body fat for Captain America. His whole body exploded; his biceps, chest, back and legs all got massive through lots of hard work and tons of food.

The Workout

Evans stated that prior to the start of filming, he worked out for 3 months doing 2-hour workouts, sometimes twice per day. During production his workouts were much shorter but he still trained. Because his character did a lot of running during the shoot, Evans was sprinting in full garb throughout the day. He had to be able to recover from a 100-meter sprint as quickly as possible to not slow down filming.

Part of Evans' workouts were bodyweight exercises such as pull-ups and push-ups. As he got bigger and stronger, his trainer strapped a weight vest on his back or extra weight from a weight belt on his hips to force him to stay In the 12–15 rep range for 3 sets. This method will make you bigger and stronger, as opposed to adding more reps, which becomes more about endurance over 15 reps. Waterson would add a few pounds periodically to keep Evans in that range and over time Evans worked up to using 33 pounds of external weight while doing pull-ups and 66 pounds in dips, not to mention the added weight of his bigger body!

Monday (a.m.)			Conditioning Circuit		
	Sets	Reps	Time/Tempo	Rest	Notes
1a) Burpees & Pull-ups	5		30	15	
1b) 2-Hand Swings	5		30	15	
1c) Step-Downs & Squat Thrusts	5		30	15	
1d) Reverse Flyes on Suspension Trainer	5		30	15	
1e) Thrusters	5		30	15	
1 minute rest between circuits					
Monday (p.m.)			Back & Arms		
1a) Deadlifts	5	8–10		minimal rest between exercises	circuit
1b) Shrugs	5	10–12			
1c) Barbell Curls	5	10–12			
1d) Pull-Ups	5	AMRAP			
Tuesday			Cardio & Abs		
1) Sprint/Jog Intervals	12		5 sec	30 sec	
5 minutes rest					
2) Hanging Leg Raises	1	AMRAP			
3) Plank or Plank & Reach	1		2-minute hold OR 50 reps		
4) Side Plank	1		at least 90 sec each side		
5) Unicycles	1		30 sec R, 30 sec L		
6) Walkouts/Ab Rollouts	1		AMRAP		

Wednesday (a.m.)	Conditioning Circuit				
	Sets	*Reps*	*Time/Tempo*	*Rest*	*Notes*
1a) Burpees & Pull-Ups	5		30	15	
1b) 2-Hand Swing	5		30	15	
1c) Step-Downs & Squat Thrusts	5		30	15	
1d) Reverse Flyes on Suspension Trainer	5		30	15	
1e) Thrusters	5		30	15	
1 minute rest between circuits					
Wednesday (p.m.)	Complete all the sets of one lift before moving to the next. You're resting 4 minutes after the squat set and after the weighted lunge set.				
1) Power Cleans	4	6–8		1 min	
2) Barbell Back Squats	5	6–8		2 min	
2 minutes rest					
3) Weighted Lunges	5	6–8		2 min	
2 minutes rest					
4) Weighted Step-Ups	5	6–8		2 min	
Thursday	Cardio & Abs				
1) Sprint/Jog Intervals	12		5 sec	30 sec	
5 minutes rest					
2) Hanging Leg Raises	1	AMRAP			
3) Plank or Plank & Reach	1		2-minute hold OR 50 reps		
4) Side Plank	1		at least 90 sec each side		
5) Unicycles	1		30 sec R, 30 sec L		
6) Walkouts/Ab Rollouts	1		AMRAP		

Friday	Conditioning Circuit				
	Sets	*Reps*	*Time/Tempo*	*Rest*	*Notes*
1a) Burpees & Pull-Ups	5		30	15	
1b) 2-Hand Swings	5		30	15	
1c) Step-Downs & Squat Thrusts	5		30	15	
1d) Reverse Flyes on Suspension Trainer	5		30	15	
1e) Thrusters	5		30	15	
1 minute rest between circuits					
Friday	Chest, Arms, Shoulders				
1a) Bench Presses	5	8		minimal rest between exercises	superset: do A followed by D, continuing until you've finished all sets of each; minimal rest between exercises
1b) ½ Kneeling DB/KB Presses	5	8			
2 minutes rest					
2a) Close-Grip Incline Bench Presses	4	10			
2b) Dips	4	10			
2 minutes rest					
3a) Triangle Push-Ups	4	AMRAP			superset
3b) Dumbbell Flyes	4	10			
Saturday	Active Recovery: moderate walk, swimming, yoga, etc.				

CHRIS HEMSWORTH
WORKOUT APPROACH FOR
THOR

A 6'3" surfer dude born in Australia and raised in the Outback, Chris Hemsworth played Captain Kirk's father, George, in the opening of the 2009 *Star Trek* film. He's perhaps best known for his role as Thor in the 2011 flick of the same name. Funnily, Hemsworth had to compete against his brother Liam for the part. Hemsworth also revived the Thor role in *The Avengers*.

Although he was in shape, Hemsworth weighed around 185 pounds and supposedly never lifted weights before getting the role of Thor. Through his training and diet, he supposedly put on about 20 pounds of muscle in just a few months, which is amazing. While it's true that beginning weightlifters can make some pretty fast gains, usually you're looking at 5–8 pounds in a few months, not 20.

The Workout

Eric Cressey, an experienced fitness professional from Massachusetts, put the following routine together for *Men's Health* magazine. This isn't what Hemsworth did to train, but it's a good fat-burning circuit that trains actions similar to using Thor's hammer. Hemsworth was reportedly too big and needed to lose some weight for filming. This workout would've worked well.

For this workout you'll perform 8 reps on each side for the first 3 exercises, and 15 reps per leg for the fourth. Go through all reps of all exercises with no rest. Rest 1 minute after completing the circuit and repeat 3 more times.

	Sets	Reps	Rest
Sledgehammers (to a tire or big block of wood)	4	8	0
Lateral Hops	4	8	0
T Push-Ups	4	8	0
Mountain Climbers	4	30	1 min

* * *

To bulk him up, Hemsworth's trainer Michael Knight created a bodybuilding type of workout, working the chest and back one day, legs on the second day and arms on the third day. He varied the program weekly by changing the number of reps; the rest between exercises was kept to a minimum and was no more than 2 minutes between supersets.

Monday	Chest & Back			
	Weeks 1, 4 & 7	*Weeks 2, 5 & 8*	*Week 3 & 6*	*Rest*
1a) Bench Presses	4 sets 4–6 reps	4 sets 6–8 reps	4 sets 8–12 reps	minimal
1b) Bent-Over Rows	4 sets 4–6 reps	4 sets 6–8 reps	4 sets 8–12 reps	minimal
2 minutes rest				
2a) Weighted Pull-Ups	4 sets 4–6 reps	4 sets 6–8 reps	4 sets 8–12 reps	minimal
2b) Weighted Dips	4 sets 4–6 reps	4 sets 6–8 reps	4 sets 8–12 reps	minimal
Wednesday	Legs			
	Weeks 1, 4 & 7	*Weeks 2, 5 & 8*	*Week 3 & 6*	*Rest*
1a) Squats	4 sets 4–6 reps	4 sets 6–8 reps	4 sets 8–12 reps	minimal
1b) Deadlifts	4 sets 4–6 reps	4 sets 6–8 reps	4 sets 8–12 reps	minimal
1c) Hamstring Curls w/ stability ball or suspension system	4 sets 4–6 reps	4 sets 6–8 reps	4 sets 8–12 reps	minimal
Friday	Arms			
	Weeks 1, 4 & 7	*Weeks 2, 5 & 8*	*Week 3 & 6*	*Rest*
1a) Weighted Chin-Ups	4 sets 4–6 reps	4 sets 6–8 reps	4 sets 8–12 reps	minimal
1b) Close-Grip Bench Presses	4 sets 4–6 reps	4 sets 6–8 reps	4 sets 8–12 reps	minimal

When the director decided Hemsworth had put on too much weight, Hemsworth had to cut way back on the building and spend more time on metabolic conditioning work to strip off excess fat. This is a conditioning workout that was added on to the main workout or done on off days.

After main workout or on separate days	Sets	Reps	Time/Tempo	Rest
1) Double KB Front Squats	8	AMRAP	20	10
1 minute rest after completing the full cycle				
2) KB Snatches (switch arms each set)	8	AMRAP	20	10
1 minute rest after completing the full cycle				
3a) 2-Hand Swings	1	AMRAP	30 sec	no rest
3b) 1-Hand Swings R	1	AMRAP	30 sec	no rest
3c) 1-Hand Swings L	1	AMRAP	30 sec	no rest
3d) H2H Swings	1	AMRAP	30 sec	1 min
4) Alternating KB Cleans (2 bells)	1	AMRAP	60 sec	1 min
5) Kettlebell Get-Ups (switch hands after each rep)	1	AMRAP	5 min	2 min
6) Kettlebell Windmills	1	5 R/L		

HUGH JACKMAN
WORKOUT APPROACH FOR
WOLVERINE

Hugh Jackman has played many different roles, from vampire-hunting Van Helsing to time-traveling, Victorian-era Englishman Leopold. He also starred with John Travolta in *Swordfish* along with Halle Barry, with whom he has worked in several of the *X-Men* movies. He is probably best-known for his character Wolverine.

With his razor-sharp claws, harder-than-steel bones, and self-healing body, Wolverine was a formidable foe and Jackman trained hard to look the part, since at 6'2" and 180 he isn't what most people consider big. His director in *X-Men Origins: Wolverine* thought Jackman looked too thin in long shots and decided Jackman needed to put on serious muscle mass so he'd look more like the comic book version, described as short and stocky. Jackman was also purportedly on a 6000-calorie diet. He went from 180 pounds to about 215 by following muscle-building workouts similar to Christian Bale's (see page 20).

As a child, Jackman played rugby and soccer, giving him an athletic background that helped him tremendously when playing action roles. He has also done dance and yoga and even appeared on the September 19, 2011, edition of *WWE Raw*, helping Zack Ryder defeat Dolph Ziggler.

The Workouts

In order to have Jackman's Wolverine match the descriptions in the comic book, Jackman did lots of strength work in the 3–5 rep range, along with more traditional bodybuilding workouts in the 8–10 rep range. These bodybuilding workouts focused on the chest, back and legs—specifically squats and deadlifts to work the front and back sides of the lower body. Jackman also did some conditioning work to make sure he didn't add any fat to his body.

The following are the exercises Jackman supposedly did to prepare for *X Men Origins: Wolverine*. Jackman's trainer Mike Ryan used the superset concept, where you perform one exercise then immediately perform another that (usually) uses the opposite muscles from the first. There's very little rest, which lets you get more work done in less time. This makes the workouts go much more quickly while still using heavy weights. Because there's very little rest, your cardiovascular system gets pushed hard too.

The weights used for each exercise should make it tough to complete each set. While you should still be able to complete each set with good form, you shouldn't be able to go more than 2 reps above what's specified.

The numbers in the Time/Tempo column refer to the speed of the lift. Typically focus on doing the eccentric portion more slowly. For example, in the bench press, slowly lower the bar to your chest for 3 counts then explode the weight up for 1 count and hold at the top for 1 count before lowering it again. This will make your muscles huge.

Monday	Chest & Triceps					
	Sets (Week 1)	Reps (Week 1)	Sets (Week 2)	Reps (Week 2)	Time/Tempo	Rest
1a) Incline DB Bench Presses	4	10–12	5	4–6	1-1-3	
1b) Dumbbell Flyes	4	10–12	5	4–6		minimal rest between exercises
2 minutes rest						
2a) Feet-Up Bench Presses	4	10–12	5	4–6	1-1-3	
2b) Cable Press-Downs	4	10–12				minimal rest between exercises
2 minutes rest						
3) Cable Crossovers	2	10–12	5	4–6		1 min
*Conditioning: Treadmill Hill Climbs	sprint 10 sec, jog 20 seconds		sprint 20 sec, jog 10 seconds		repeat for 20 min	

*Other conditioning could be:

1) Mountain climber intervals: 20 seconds of work, 10 seconds of rest, for 4 minutes.

2) Squat jumps for 20 seconds, then regular squats for 20 seconds, then hold the bottom position of your squat for 20 seconds. Rest 1 minute and repeat for a total of 3 to 5 sets.

3) Max-effort sprints in intervals of 5 seconds of work, 30 seconds of rest, for 8–10 minutes. As these get easier, shorten the rest period by 5 seconds. Work toward 15 seconds of work and 15 seconds of rest for 8 rounds.

Tuesday	Legs					
	Sets (Week 1)	*Reps (Week 1)*	*Sets (Week 2)*	*Reps (Week 2)*	*Time/Tempo*	*Rest*
1a) Barbell Back Squats	4	10–12	5	4–6	3-0-1	
1b) Dumbbell Rear Foot Elevated Split Squats	4	10–12 per leg	5	4–6 per leg	3-0-1	minimal rest between exercises
	2 minutes rest					
2a) Romanian Deadlifts	4	10–12	5	4–6	3-1-1	
2b) 1-Leg Stability Ball Hamstring Curls	4	10–12 per leg	5	4–6 per leg	3-1-3	minimal rest between exercises
	2 minutes rest					
3) Walking DB Lunges	2	to exhaustion	2	to exhaustion		1 min
Conditioning: Rowing Machine	1	*4000m (2.5 miles)	1	4000m (2.5 miles)		

*Cover the 4000 meters by sprinting then dropping back to a normal pace every 15 seconds. If you don't have a rowing machine, it'll be tough to duplicate this work, which is very back- and leg-intensive and also strengthens the core.

Wednesday	Rest: do some stretching or a light bodyweight workout.

Thursday	Back & Biceps					
1a) Cable Rows w/ resistance band, KB or DB	4	10	5	4–6	3-1-2	minimal rest between exercises
1b) Bent-Over DB Reverse Flyes	4	10	5	4–6		
	2 minutes rest					
2a) Neutral-Grip Chin-Ups	4	10	5	4–6	1-1-2	
2b) EZ-Bar Curls	4	10	5	4–6	2-1-3	minimal rest between exercises
	2 minutes rest					
Inverted Rows	2	AMRAP	2	AMRAP	3-1-2	1 min
Conditioning: Bike Sprint Intervals					10 sec work, 50 sec rest for 4–6 min	

Friday			Shoulders & Abdominals			
	Sets (Week 1)	Reps (Week 1)	Sets (Week 2)	Reps (Week 2)	Time/Tempo	Rest
1a) Seated DB Overhead Presses	4	10 R/L	5	4–6 R/L	2-1-2	minimal rest between exercises
1b) Dumbbell Lateral Raises	4	10	5	4–6		
2 minutes rest						
2a) L1–Walkouts L2–Stability Ball Rollouts L3–Ab Rollouts (on knees) L4–Ab Rollouts (standing)	4	AMRAP	5	AMRAP		minimal rest between exercises
2b) Stability Ball Jack Knives	4	AMRAP	5	AMRAP		
2 minutes rest						
Unicycles	4		6		30 sec R/L	15 sec
Conditioning: Treadmill Intervals	10		10		sprint 5 sec, jog 30 sec	

BRUCE LEE
WORKOUT APPROACH

Bruce Lee is the ultimate martial artist—incredibly ripped, fast and powerful. Although he was about 5'7" and weighed roughly 145 pounds soaking wet, he could send you flying with his patented 1-inch punch. He routinely kicked a 300-pound bag so hard it would slam the ceiling. Lee probably had about 5% body fat—you could see every muscle in his body with every movement he made.

Lee's first major U.S. role was as Kato in the mid-1960s TV series *The Green Hornet*. The Green Hornet was a counter to Batman, and both Bruce Lee and Van William (who played the Green Hornet as well as media mogul and playboy Britt Reid) appeared in several episodes of *Batman*. *The Green Hornet* only ran for one season, but it made Lee a star in the U.S. Back home in Hong Kong, the show was so popular they called it *The Kato Show*.

After *The Green Hornet,* Lee went on to star in major martial arts flicks, bringing a more realistic sense to them as opposed to some of the more esoteric kung fu movies made in China, many of which were based on Chinese legends. Lee's first big U.S. movie was *Fists of Fury* (originally called *Big Boss*) and he appeared in four episodes of the TV show *Longstreet*. Two of Lee's martial arts students (actor James Coburn and script writer Stirling Silliphant) helped Bruce create *The Silent Flute*, a film that was never finished but formed the basis for the David Carradine movie *Circle of Iron*. Lee's most popular movie was *Enter the Dragon*, which he wrote, choreographed and starred in. He died just before it was released.

The concept for the 1970s TV show *Kung Fu*, which starred Carradine as Kwai Chang Caine, was also created by Lee, but he was never given credit for it. The studio said they had a similar story line that was developed independently and they wouldn't let Lee play the lead because of his thick accent.

The Workout

Lee was naturally lean but built his body with years of hard work. He spent countless hours lifting weights, running, hitting the heavy bag, and practicing and teaching Jeet Kune Do, the system he created by taking the best techniques from all the other martial arts. He's considered by many to be the first mixed martial artist (MMA), borrowing from jujitsu, karate, kung fu, savate (French), and Indonesian and Filipino martial arts. To detail Lee's exact training would require several books dedicated to his training. For more information, see his book *Tao of Jeet Kune Do*.

In short, Lee's routine included kettlebells, barbells and other equipment, and he did squats, bench presses, swings, push-ups and many other full-body exercises. He had performed a lot of bodybuilding-type lifting that focused on muscle isolation, but he found it made him tight, slowed him down and took away from his power so he switched to more full-body work.

Lee recognized that it's better to train hard but not to fatigue. If you train to failure or exhaustion, you won't be able to function at peak efficiency if the need arises. For Lee, this meant he had to be able to fight at any time. What brought this concept home to him was an incident that occurred shortly after he opened a martial arts school in the U.S. At that time the Chinese weren't supposed to teach their arts to non-Chinese people. Lee disagreed with this and felt that everyone should have the opportunity to learn Chinese martial arts.

When another master tried to shut Lee's school down, Lee had to fight off the master and several of his students. Lee won but the fight (which only lasted about 4 minutes) left him very winded and tired. He realized he'd have to be smarter about his training and improve his conditioning and strength—all without leaving him too tired to fight if he had to.

This same concept should be used by everyone today, especially first responders—lives may depend on it. Consider a cop who goes to the gym and lifts so heavy he can barely move or trains to failure. If he then has to go on duty, he'll be at a distinct disadvantage if he has to chase or subdue a suspect.

John Saxon, an actor (he played Roper in *Enter the Dragon*) and Lee's student, stated in an interview that Lee had a weight set that included handles on which plates were loaded. These handles allowed Lee to do swings, which are a great exercise for developing hip snap (the hip snap is where the power for a punch comes from). Saxon and Dan Inosanto, another student of Lee's and now the head of the Jeet Kune Do system, both train with kettlebells, having learned from Pavel Tsatsouline.

In addition to weight training, Lee practiced isometric, or static, holds against his own body and weights. Basically, you tighten up and resist your own movement, say a punch, or hold a weight for as long as possible without moving. This helps build tendon and ligament strength, which is actually more important than muscle strength. Tendons attach muscle to bone and ligaments hold bones together. A muscle that's too strong for its tendon or the ligaments around it can tear that connective tissue, sometimes completely from the bone! The drawback to doing isometric holds is you only get strong in the position that you hold. Another way to strengthen connective tissue is to do ballistic movements like those done using a kettlebell: swings, cleans and snatches.

Lee also made sure he stretched out after his weight-training sessions so that he didn't get tight and lose his flexibility. You should always stretch at the end of every workout as part of a total fitness regime. You also need to do activation and mobilization of the muscles and joints before working out to properly prepare the body for the work it's about to do.

WORKOUT 1

The following workout is from www. mikementzer.com/blee.html. This is just one of many routines that Lee did over the course of his short life. Done as a circuit, it's a very good basic workout and can be performed 2

to 3 days per week. We've added in deadlifts and some kettlebell work to target the hamstrings and glutes more. For example: Do 2x20 kettlebell swings as a warm-up before doing the main workout, then do 2x8 deadlifts after the barbell curls.

After 4 weeks you should switch to a different routine. The body adapts to a stimulus in about 4 weeks, so by changing up the workout you'll continue to see gains. Also each week try to go up in weight but make sure you aren't training to failure.

Exercise	Sets	Reps
Clean & Press	2	8
Squats	2	12
Dumbbell Pullovers	2	8
Bench Presses	2	6
Good Mornings	2	8
Barbell Curls	2	8

WORKOUT 2

Lee did a lot of ab work:

- Waist Twists—4 sets of 90 reps
- Sit-Up Twists—4 sets of 20 reps
- Leg Raises—4 sets of 20 reps
- Leaning Twists—4 sets of 50 reps
- Frog Kicks—4 sets of 50 reps

He also liked:

- Roman Chair Sit-Ups
- Side Bends

Recent studies by Dr. Stuart McGill of the University of Waterloo in Ontario,

Canada, one of the top spine researchers in the world, have shown that doing sit-ups, crunches and twisting from the lower back puts tremendous loads on the discs and he recommends against doing this type of work as it will wear out the lower back. Instead, focus on stabilizing the torso and preventing rotation.

Instead of the above, do this workout. Perform the planks then the side planks with no rest in between, then do the other exercises as a circuit.

	Sets	Reps	Time/Tempo	Rest	Notes
Plank Hold	1		2 min minimum		strict form!
Side Plank	1		90 sec R/L	1 min	
Bird Dog	3	5 R/L	2-5-2		
Dead Bug	3		30 sec		
Heavy Band/Cable Pallof Presses	3	8 R/L	3-1-3		
Low Windmills	3	6 R/L	3-0-3		
Kettlebell Renegade Rows	3	10 R/L			
Super Plank	3	10			
Walkouts or Stability Ball or Ab Rollouts	3	10			
Leg Raises	3	10		1 min	

BRAD PITT
WORKOUT APPROACH FOR
FIGHT CLUB, SNATCH, TROY

At 5'11½" and roughly 155 pounds, Brad Pitt was at 5–6% body fat for his role as Tyler Durden in the film *Fight Club*. He was extremely lean—5–6% body fat is very hard to achieve as well as difficult to maintain for more than a few months. Many guys went crazy trying to lean out like Pitt but most didn't do what needed to be done. The secret wasn't in the workouts he did but in how he ate. Nutrition is 80–90% of how you look and how much body fat you carry. You can exercise until the cows come home but without proper nutrition you'll never get the best results possible.

As a teenager Pitt grew up playing golf and tennis and was on the swim and wrestling teams, which provided him with a well-rounded athletic background. When he was preparing for *Fight Club*, he studied boxing, taekwondo and grappling (probably jujitsu or Brazilian jujitsu).

Right after *Fight Club*, Pitt was in the British movie *Snatch*, in which he played an Irish boxer with a very thick, almost unintelligible accent. For this role his physique changed a little as he ate more normally, put on some muscle and went up to about 8% body fat. After *Snatch* he starred in several other movies, including *The Mexican* with Julia Roberts and *Ocean's Eleven*. His physique wasn't as much of a factor until he played Achilles in *Troy*.

Many people have pointed out that he gained 20 pounds for *Troy* versus his weight in *Snatch* and they make it sound as though these two movies were done close together when in fact four years separated them. He supposedly started training six or seven months before filming began and it's unclear what his physique was like beforehand. Gaining 20–25 pounds and staying around 8% body fat would be tough but not impossible, especially when taking into account his diet of lean meats, veggies and protein shakes; he had also stopped smoking and gave up junk food like chips and beer.

The Workouts

Pitt's workouts for *Snatch* and *Fight Club* were exclusively upper body workouts and you can see it in the build of his lower body; his quads, thighs and calves are underdeveloped in comparison to his upper body. In contrast, his *Troy* workouts had squats, deadlifts and other lower body work but, still, most of his workout was focused on upper body bulking. We made some tweaks to both workouts so you won't neglect your lower body as Pitt did.

Since Pitt was already in pretty good shape before *Fight Club,* his workouts for *Fight Club* and *Snatch* focused on getting him stronger and leaner. His *Troy* workouts were geared more toward piling muscle on his very lean frame without adding fat.

Pitt worked out 5 days per week, with weight training Monday through Thursday and cardio on Friday. Saturday and Sunday were rest/recovery days. Most of the weight training was probably done in the 12–15 rep range with a light to moderate weight, with 60 seconds of rest between sets.

FIGHT CLUB/SNATCH WORKOUT

Pitt's original workout has no leg training at all and is very unbalanced. The back work is all upper back, neglecting the more important muscles of the lower back, which act as stabilizers along with the abs. We propose a more balanced approach to get the same look as Pitt without the drawbacks.

Monday	Chest & Back				
	Sets	Reps	Time/Tempo	Rest	Notes
1a) Push-Ups	1	AMRAP			superset: do A followed by B, continuing until you've finished all sets of each
1b) Pull-Ups	1	AMRAP		2 min	
					choose a push-up variation that's challenging to you
2a) Bench Presses	3	10–12			superset
2b) Bent Rows	3	10–12		1 min	
2 minutes rest					
3) Dumbbell Flyes	3	10		1 min	
Tuesday	**Legs**				
1a) Deadlifts	3	10–12		30 sec	superset
1b) Rear Foot Elevated Split Squats	3	10 R/L		2 min	
2 minutes rest					
2a) Front Squats	3	10–12		30 sec	superset • go heavy
2b) 2-Hand KB Swings	3	10–12		2 min	
1 minute rest					
3) Calf Raises	3	12–15		60 sec–90 sec	
Wednesday	**Arms & Abs**				
1a) Barbell Curls	3	10–12	2-1-2		superset
1b) Triceps Extensions	3	8–10	2-1-2		
3 minutes rest					
2a) EZ-Bar Curls	3	10–12	2-1-2		superset
2b) Triceps Kickbacks	3	10 R/L	2-1-2		
3) Hanging Leg Raises	1	AMRAP			
1 minute rest					
4) Unicycles	3		30 sec R/L	30 sec	

Thursday			Shoulders		
	Sets	Reps	Time/Tempo	Rest	Notes
1a) Overhead Presses	3	8–10			superset
1b) Shoulder Shrugs	3	15–20			
2 minutes rest					
2a) Reverse Flyes	3	10–12			superset
2b) Upright Rows	3	10–12		2 min	
Friday			Boxing, Fight Training, HIIT		
Sprint	4–5		3–5 seconds	6–30 sec	all out
OR					
1a) Squat Thrusts	5		15 sec	15 sec	tri-set
1b) 2-Hand KB Swings	5		15 sec	15 sec	
1c) Super Plank	5		15 sec	15 sec	
Saturday			Rest: do some stretching or a light bodyweight workout.		
Sunday			Rest: do some stretching or a light bodyweight workout.		

TROY WORKOUT

The *Troy* workout is more balanced than the *Fight Club/Snatch* workout. Since this is a bodybuilding routine, complete all the sets and reps of one exercise before moving to the next. Normally we prefer working in super- or tri-sets but this would mean a major re-write of this program to be able to work it in that manner.

Monday			Chest		
	Sets	Reps	Time/Tempo	Rest	Notes
Bench Presses	5	6–10		3 min	
Incline Bench Presses	6	6–10		3 min	
Cable Crossovers	6	10–12		3 min	
Dips	5	AMRAP		3 min	
Dumbbell Pullovers	5	10–12		3 min	

Tuesday	Back & Legs				
	Sets	Reps	Time/Tempo	Rest	Notes
Wide-Grip Chin-Ups	6	AMRAP		2 min	
T-Bar Rows	6	6–10		3 min	
Seated Pulley Rows	6	10–12		3 min	
Romanian Deadlift	5	15		3 min	
Squats	6	8–12		3 min	
Leg Presses	6	8–12			
Leg Extensions	6	12–15			
Barbell Lunges	5	15			
Wednesday	**Calves & Forearms**				
Standing Calf Raises	10	10			
Seated Calf Raises	8	15			
1-Leg Calf Raises (holding dumbbells)	6	12 R/L			
Wrist Curls (forearms on knees)	4	10			
Barbell Reverse Wrist Curls	4	8			
Wrist Rollers	1	AMRAP			
Thursday	**Biceps & Triceps**				
Barbell Curls	6	6–10			
Seated DB Curls	6	6–10			
Dumbbell Concentration Curls	6	6–10			
Close-Grip Bench Presses	6	6–10			
Press-Downs	6	6–10			
Barbell French Presses	6	6–10			
1-Arm DB Triceps Extensions	6	6–10			

Friday			Shoulders & Abs		
	Sets	Reps	Time/Tempo	Rest	Notes
Seated Barbell Presses	6	6–10			
Standing Lateral Raises	6	6–10			
Rear Lateral Raises	6	6–10			
Cable Lateral Raises	5	10–12			
2 minutes rest					
1a) Plank	3		2–5 min		strict form
1b) Side Plank	3		60–90 sec R/L	30 sec	
30 seconds rest					
2a) Unicycles			30 sec R/L		
2b) Hanging Knee or Leg Raises	5	AMRAP		30 sec	
30 seconds rest					
3) Mountain Climbers	8		20 sec	10 sec	
Saturday	Rest: do some stretching or a light bodyweight workout.				
Sunday	Rest: do some stretching or a light bodyweight workout.				

ANDY WHITFIELD
WORKOUT APPROACH FOR
SPARTACUS

Welsh actor Andy Whitfield played the lead role in the Starz TV series *Spartacus*. The show was loosely based on an ancient Thracian who was either a captured Greek soldier or a slave in service to the Romans. It's known that Spartacus trained at the Roman gladiatorial school and managed to escape with about 70 others. Whitfield was extremely lean, strong and athletic—he epitomized the Greek warrior look and looked like he could move well and fight to the death.

The Workout

Before filming started, Whitfield and the other *Spartacus* actors spent about a month at "Gladiator Camp," where they trained for 4 hours every morning. Part of that training worked on the actors' overall athleticism. They practiced diving, rolling, tumbling and general fight training, weapons maneuvers and martial arts–specific exercises. The camp also put them through grueling circuit-style workouts that were similar to those done by the actors in the film *300*. They did lots of tire flipping, sledgehammer work, deadlifts, pull-ups, dips, kettlebell lifts, curls and more. They also performed a lot of cardio work on rowing machines to both build their back muscles and increase their conditioning levels even more.

Men's Health magazine created two different workouts that they dubbed Spartacus and Spartacus 2.0. However, neither of these were actually done by the actors to prepare for the roles.

SPARTACUS

This extremely challenging workout consists of 10 full-body exercises done for 60 seconds each with a 15-second break between exercises. Go through this circuit 3 times with a 2-minute rest after completing each circuit. You'll need a couple of dumbbells or kettlebells. The weight should be such that you're challenged for 15 to 20 reps. If you can't do the full minute at each station, do the best you can. After doing the workout a few times you'll be able to get through it as written.

Do this workout 3 times per week for a month and you'll be in the best shape of your life and look like a Greek warrior.

EXERCISES

- Goblet Squats
- Mountain Climbers
- 1-Hand Dumbbell Swings
- Dumbbell T Push-Ups (use hex dumbbells so they can't roll)
- Jumping Lunges
- Dumbbell Bent Rows
- Dumbbell Side Lunge & Touch
- Dumbbell Renegade Rows
- Dumbbell Lunge and Rotation
- Dumbbell Push Presses

SPARTACUS WORKOUT 2.0

This workout requires 40 seconds of work and 20 seconds of rest. There are two 5-exercise circuits. Do Circuit 1 twice without a break in between, then rest 2 minutes and repeat the circuit twice more. After completing Circuit 1 a total of 4 times, rest 2 minutes and move to Circuit 2, which will be done the same way as Circuit 1: Do it twice, rest 2 minutes, then do it 2 more times. For exercises done on one side, switch sides each circuit; don't do both sides in the same cycle. For example, for the 1-hand swing, do it on the right side the first time through the circuit, then do the left arm the second time through.

CIRCUIT 1

- Dumbbell Hang Pulls
- Offset Lunges (dumbbell held at shoulder height)
- 1-Hand Swings (dumbbell or kettlebell)
- Thrusters
- 1-Leg, 1-Arm, Underhand-Grip Dumbbell Rows

CIRCUIT 2

- Dumbbell Wood Chops
- Super Plank
- Rotational 1-Leg Straight-Leg Deadlifts
- Squat Thrusts
- Jump Squats

If you have access to a heavy tire and a sledgehammer, you can create a challenging "finisher" to do after the main workout or on a separate day:

1 Hit the tire with the sledgehammer 25 times with your right hand lead and then 25 times with your left lead.   **2** Flip the tire 50 feet, run back and get the sledgehammer, run back to the tire and do 25 more hits with the sledgehammer on each side.   **3** Flip the tire back to the start. Run back and get the sledgehammer and repeat until you're toasty.

PART 3: EXERCISES

PRESSES

Barbell Bench Press

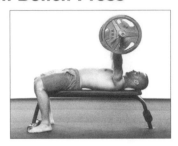

1 With the bar on the uprights of the bench and loaded with the appropriate weight (use collars to lock the plates in place), position yourself face up on the bench so that your shoulders are even with or slightly below the uprights. Place your hands a little wider than your shoulders on the bar and have your spotter help you get the bar off the uprights. Your feet should be flat on the floor. If they aren't, put a plate or 2 under each foot. Squeeze the bar. **2** Press from your lats and straighten your elbows. Pause at the top and slowly bring the bar back to your chest.

Close-Grip Bench Press

Bring the hands closer together to work the triceps more.

Incline Bench Press

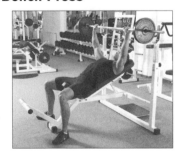

Elevate the bench to the desired angle and perform a bench press.

Close-Grip Incline Bench Press

Bring the hands closer together to work the triceps more.

Kettlebell Floor Press

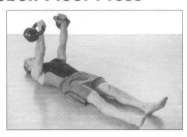

1 Lie on your back and get your kettlebells into position. Keep your elbows bent 90 degrees, your triceps on the ground and your forearms perpendicular to the floor; the bells should be on the backs of your forearms. **2** Press the weight up, focusing on your lats. Lock out your elbows. Your hands should still be in line with your chest or slightly below. **3** To bring the bells down, PULL them as though someone were holding them, preventing you from getting them back down.

Single Kettlebell Floor Press

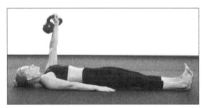

Pull one kettlebell down and press it back up repeatedly for the allotted time interval. Then switch sides. This is one set.

Dumbbell Floor Press

A floor press can also be done with dumbbells.

Barbell Floor Press

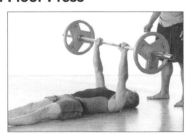

A floor press can also be done with a barbell.

Band Chest Press

1 Securely attach a band to a door or post and then step away from the post, facing away. Position the band across your palm so that both sides of the band are inside your arm. The hand should be slightly forward of your ribs and about even with the bottom 2 ribs. There should be no slack in the band at the start position. Make sure the band is perpendicular to the post and you. If you're too far to one side, it'll rub against your ribs or shirt. Keep your elbow close to your body. **2** Staying tight and avoiding any upper body rotation, extend your arm straight out about chest height.

There are several ways to stand:

Even Stance Band Chest Press

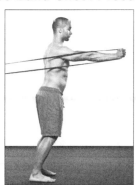

Step your feet about shoulder-width apart. You'll be leaning forward slightly from your ankles to keep the band from pulling you back. Don't allow your waist or hips to bend.

Staggered Stance Band Chest Press

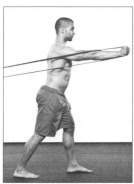

Step one foot forward of the other about a natural step apart; bend the front knee. Feet are hip-width apart and point forward. Typically you'll press from the back-foot side of the body and switch feet when you switch hands.

Tall Kneeling Band Chest Press

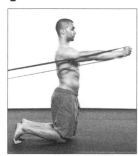

You may want a yoga mat or something similar to pad your knees. Kneel down with both knees on the floor so that they're not touching each other. Your thighs should be vertical front and side. Squeeze your glutes and keep your hips under you as you press. You should feel your abs and glutes kick in hard to keep you from falling over.

Half Kneeling Band Chest Press

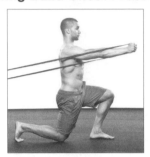

Place one knee on the floor and step the other foot in front of you, bending the knee 90 degrees. The front shin and back thigh are vertical; you should be on the ball of the rear foot. Stay tight and squeeze your glutes, keeping your hips under you as you press. Typically you'll press from the same side as the down knee.

Band Punches

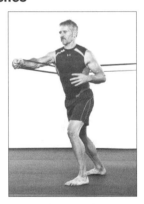

This is the same as a band chest press (page 81) but fast and explosive, using hip rotation to create power. You can either punch with a vertical fist, palm facing inward, or a traditional "reverse" punch where you rotate the arm so that the palm is face down when the arm is extended.

1 Just like throwing a punch, explode one arm forward, rotating through your feet and hips. Keep the elbow close to your side. **2** Let the band/arm come back to your side, turning at the hips and feet a little beyond the start position.

Make sure to do both sides.

OVERHEAD PRESSES

Band Overhead Press

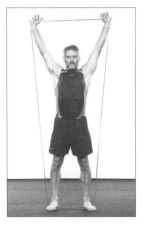

1 Stand inside a band with your feet hip-width apart so that the band is under the mid-part of each foot. Hold an end of the band in each hand with the band crossing the palms. Your hands should be just wider than your shoulders. To adjust the tension of the band, create slack between your feet to make it hard to press or remove slack from between your feet to make it easier. **2** Drive your hands up and slightly wider than the start position. Lock your elbows but don't hyperextend them.

Kettlebell Overhead Press

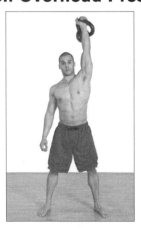

1 Clean the kettlebell and hold it in rack position. Move your feet under your hips and grab the ground with your toes. Squeeze your armpit so your lat touches your triceps. You'll now either: **a.** Press the bell straight up by squeezing everything tightly and keeping the movement slow and controlled. Keep your forearm vertical and your elbow locked throughout the movement. **b.** Move your elbow out toward your side at the same time you start to press. Keep your forearm vertical and your elbow locked. When your elbow is nearly straight, your forearm should move up and in. This is the Arnold Press.

Double Kettlebell Overhead Press

Clean 2 bells and press them both at the same time, using all the tension, breathing and movement patterns you learned on the single press.

Dumbbell Overhead Press

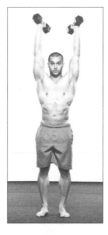

Bring 1 or 2 dumbbells to shoulder height for either press (standard or Arnold).

Push Press

This is a "cheat" version of the overhead press to let you get a heavier weight overhead. It can be done with dumbbells or kettlebells.

1 Curl 2 bells to shoulder height, keeping your elbows close to your body. **2** Keeping your torso upright, do a partial squat, folding at the hips. **3** Quickly straighten your hips and knees and press the bells straight up so your hands are over your shoulders. **4** With control, lower the bells back to shoulder level.

Half Kneeling Overhead Press

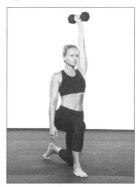

This overhead press can be done with dumbbells or kettlebells. The goal is to keep your torso from moving, bending or leaning. Place one knee on the floor and step the other foot in front of you, bending the knee 90 degrees. You should be on the ball of the rear foot, and the front leg shouldn't move out to the side. Stay tight and squeeze your glutes, keeping your hips under you as you press. Typically you'll press from the same side as the down knee.

Tall Kneeling Overhead Press

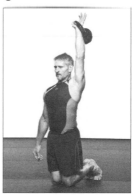

This overhead press can be done with dumbbells or kettlebells, but you'll kneel with both knees on the floor, not touching each other, and thighs perpendicular to the floor. The focus is on core stability. Keep your glutes tight and your hips under you.

Seated Overhead Press

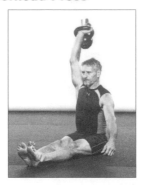

This intermediate to advanced press starts by sitting on the floor and can use kettlebells or dumbbells. Your legs should be extended straight in front of you. The farther apart your feet are from touching, the easier it is. Sit up tall when you do the press—don't lean back!

Alternating Overhead Press

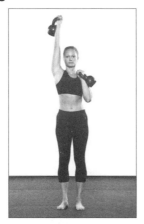

Using kettlebells or dumbbells while standing or sitting, bring both bells to rack or shoulder height. Press one bell, return it to start, then press the other and bring it back down.

Barbell Overhead Press

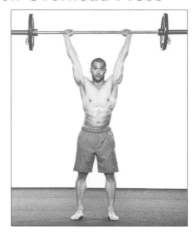

1 Clean the barbell, with the bar shoulder height and across your collar bones. Hold the bar with wrists straight or bent, palms facing forward and thumbs around the bar rather than over the top.   **2** With your feet under your hips or slightly wider, contract your body to drive the bar up. Pull your head back slightly as the bar goes up. Lock the elbows.   **3** With control, lower the bar back to your collar bones, moving your head back a little as the bar comes down.

FLYES

Dumbbell Flyes

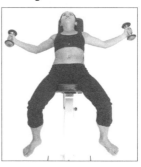

1 Lie face up on a bench (flat, inclined or declined) with a dumbbell in each hand. Keep your hands above your chest with elbows bent slightly and pointing to the sides.   **2** Keeping your elbows bent and your back on the bench, lower the dumbbells below the level of the bench or as low as you can.   **3** Bring the bells back up as if to hug someone. Stop at the top when your hands are close together but not touching.

Reverse Flye on Suspension Trainer

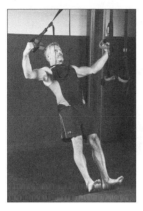

1 Adjust the suspension trainer so the handles are about shoulder height. Hold a handle in each hand with your body face up. Start with your feet under the attachment point and try to keep your knees straight. I typically keep my heels on the floor with the rest of the foot up, but you can also place your entire foot on the floor. Keep your arms extended in front of your chest, your spine in neutral, and your abs and glutes tight. **2** Bend your elbows slightly and pull your arms to the sides and a little behind you. This should make your body rise up almost upright. Stick out your chest and squeeze your shoulder blades together. If this is too hard, move your body backward a little so your torso is more upright.

PULL-APARTS

Horizontal Band Chest Pull-Apart

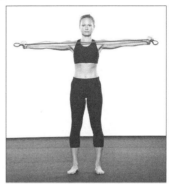

1 Hold the band in front of you with your hands at shoulder height and slightly wider than your shoulders, palms facing down. The closer together your hands are to the center of the band, the harder this is. **2** Keeping your elbows straight and squeezing everything tight, pull your shoulder blades back and move your hands directly to the sides.

Diagonal Band Chest Pull-Apart

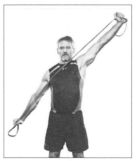

Starting with your hands the same as in the horizontal version, pull one hand high and the other low to opposite sides. Slowly return to start and repeat but switch the hand orientations.

HIGH PULLS

Barbell High Pull

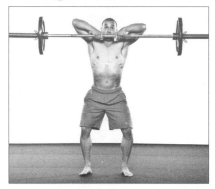

1 Stand behind a loaded barbell with your feet about shoulder-width apart. Keeping your shins close to vertical, squat down and grab the bar with your hands just inside your legs.   **2** Explode straight up with your hips. As the bar rises, use your upper back and traps to bring the bar up to just below your chin. Keep your elbows up.   **3** Then let the bar fall straight down—as it passes your midsection, squat down quickly and absorb the weight with your legs. Don't try to muscle the weight up or control it with your arms on the way down. This is a fast, explosive, fluid movement—the barbell should lightly touch the floor before you explode up again.

Band High Pull

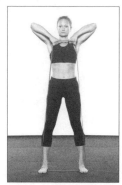

The band variations use the upper back and traps a lot more than the kettlebell and barbell versions because the resistance increases the more the band is stretched, as opposed to the bar and bell, which get "lighter" as they reach the top.

1 Stand inside the band with your feet shoulder-width apart and the band in the middle portion of each foot. Squat down and grab the top section of band and stand up until there's slight tension in the band. Your knees should still be bent and your arms straight.
2 Explode up and pull the band to your chin, keeping your elbows up.

2-Hand Kettlebell High Vertical Pull

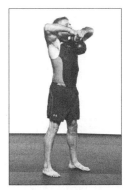

1 Step your feet shoulder-width apart and place a kettlebell between them. Squat down just enough to hold the bell with both hands, keeping your arms and wrists straight. **2** Explode straight up and use the momentum to bring the bell up, pulling minimally with your arms until the bell comes just under your chin. Keep your elbows slightly higher than your hands. **3** Let the bell fall straight down; as it passes your midsection, begin to squat. The bell should softly touch the ground, the energy being absorbed by your legs. This is a very smooth, continuous movement.

Dumbbell Hang Pull

1 Stand with your feet shoulder-width apart with a dumbbell in each hand, arms by your sides and palms facing the rear. **2** Do a partial squat and explode up while pulling the bells to just below shoulder height. Your elbows should be slightly higher than your shoulders. **3** Let the bells fall straight back to the outsides of your legs; absorb the downward energy by flexing your hips and knees.

KETTLEBELL SWINGS

2-Hand Kettlebell Swing

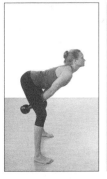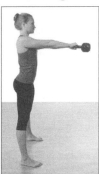

1 Stand with your feet a little wider than your shoulders. Place the bell out in front, slightly beyond your reach. Push your hips straight back and bend your knees a little. With both hands on the bell, hike it back between your legs so your forearms are in your groin. Keep your abs tight. **2** Shoot your hips straight forward and drive through your heels, simultaneously raising your torso and moving the bell in a forward arc to chin height. As the bell reaches the peak of the swing, forcefully contract your glutes, hamstrings and abs, but keep just enough tension in your arms to hold the bell. You should be standing tall with your abs tight, pelvis tucked under and elbows slightly bent. The bottom of the bell is in line with your straight wrists. **3** Reverse the movement by pushing your hips back. The arms trace their path back between your legs to the start position. Continue to keep your lats tight, chest out, shoulders down and in and wrists straight. Think about hiking the bell back behind you as far as you can, not up or down.

1-Hand Kettlebell Swing

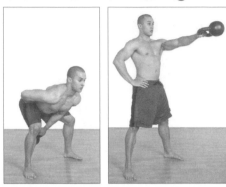

Start as you would for the 2-Hand Kettlebell Swing but place one hand on your hip or thigh. When you perform the swing, the palm of the working hand should face back and your chest should be square to the front. To avoid rotating, place the non-working hand on the wrist of the working arm. Think about hiking the bell back behind you as far as you can.

Hand-to-Hand (H2H) Kettlebell Swing

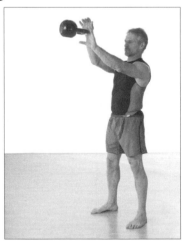

1 Perform a 1-hand swing.   **2** At the point in the swing where the bell is at its highest and just before it starts to drop, slip your free hand over the hand holding the bell and quickly pull the first hand out.

Continue the swing and hand switches.

Kettlebell Swing Flip & Squat

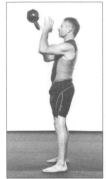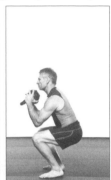

This very dynamic movement, a combination of a 2-hand swing and a goblet squat, should be fluid and non-stop.

1 Perform a 2-hand swing (page 87).   **2** As you reach the top of the swing, flick your wrists and bring your elbows in a little. The bell will rotate so that the handle will go down and around 180 degrees.   **3** Catch the ball, bring your elbows in more and squat. At this point the handle should be facing away from you.   **4** As you stand up, just before your hips lock, flip your wrists forward slightly so the bell rotates. The handle will come back under and up to the hands—catch it smoothly and move back into the swing.

Kettlebell Swing High Pull

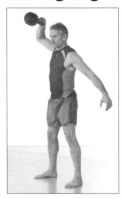

1 Perform a 1-hand swing. As the bell reaches the peak of the swing, retract your scapula while keeping your arm relaxed. Your elbow will bend as your shoulder goes back. Bring your elbow back to the side of your head until it's bent about 90 degrees, with your forearm parallel to the floor and your elbow higher than your shoulder. The bell should be in front of and slightly to the outside of your shoulder. Your hips should be locked out, and your wrist and forearm should be locked together.   **2** Quickly push the bell back out. Just as your arm straightens (don't lock your elbow), your hips should move back. Let the bell smoothly resume its normal arc back down between your legs. Make sure you push your hips back, not down, and keep the bell as far from the floor as possible. The bottom of the bell always faces out and away, never up or down, except at the bottom of the swing.

up. When your hips are fully extended, your shoulder should be at its highest point and your elbow should be higher than your shoulder.   **3** As your forearm continues upward, your elbow straightens. When your forearm approaches vertical, flip your wrist so that your fingers point up. If you're using the dead clean grip, the bell should rotate around your wrist. If you're using the 1-hand kettlebell swing grip, you'll have to be a little more aggressive with the flip or punch of the hand.

ADVANCED KETTLEBELL TECHNIQUES

Kettlebell Snatch

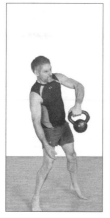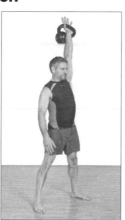

1 Place the bell on the floor between your feet as you would for dead cleans (page 94). Squat down and grab the handle with your left hand, using the dead clean grip or the 1-hand swing (page 88). Keep your torso upright and keep your elbow straight but "soft" at the start of each rep.   **2** Keeping your arm as close to your body as possible, explode straight up and pull the bell straight up off the floor. If you're using the dead clean grip (pictured), keep your thumb pointed toward you as the bell comes up. If you're using the 1-hand kettlebell swing grip, keep your palm facing you as the bell comes

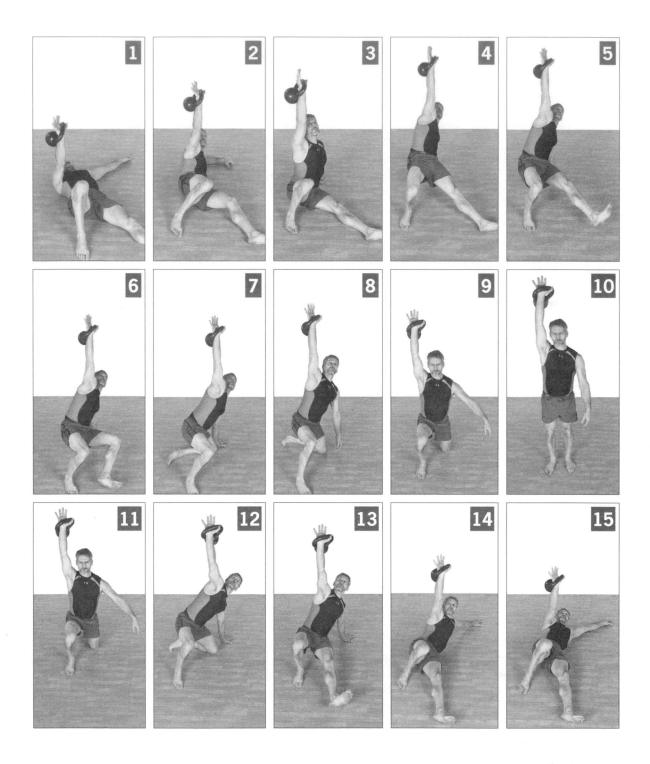

Kettlebell Turkish Get-Up

1 Lie flat on your back and press a bell with your right arm, using the same technique as the floor press (page 80). Bend your right knee to about 45 degrees with the foot flat on the floor; your left leg remains straight. Your left arm is on the floor and out to the side at shoulder level, while your right arm is locked and vertical. **2–3** Driving with your right foot, roll from your upper left arm to your elbow and forearm so that you end up with your left palm flat on the floor supporting you and almost directly under your shoulder; your torso should be upright. Your right knee is still bent and pointing up, while your left leg is straight. **4–5** Driving your right heel into the floor, lift your butt as high as you can into a bridge position. Keep your hips facing the ceiling. At the same time, drive your left shoulder into the floor by pushing the hand hard against the floor. Let your left leg rotate from the hip so that the outside edge of the foot is on the floor. **6–8** Bring your left leg under you, bending the knee and placing it just in front of your left hand. Your right shin is now close to vertical and your right foot is flat on the floor. **9** Swing your lower left leg out from under you and pivot on your knee so that your left foot is directly behind you; your torso should come up at the same time. You're now in a half kneeling position. **10** Flip onto the ball of your left foot and drive from the heel of the front foot and the ball of the back foot to a standing position. As you stand, bring your left foot forward next to your right foot. **11** To return to the floor, step back with your left foot as in a back lunge and place your left knee gently on the floor. **12** Flip your left foot so that the top of the foot is on the floor. Rotating at the hip, swing your lower left leg under you so that your toes point to the right. At the same time, push your hips to the right and place your left hand on the floor by the left knee, driving your shoulder down away from your ear. Your right knee is bent and your shin is almost vertical with your right foot, which is flat on the floor. **13** Support yourself on your left hand and flat right foot. Lift your hips and shoot your left leg out from under you, extending your knee and letting the outside of the foot rest on the floor. **14–15** Slowly slide your left arm out from under you toward the left rear. Let your

forearm then your upper arm roll to the floor. Your left side then comes into contact with the floor. Roll onto your back and into start position.

From here, you have 3 options: **1** Bring the bell down to the floor, drag it to the other side and do a rep on the left **2** leave your right arm extended and do another rep on the right **3** or re-press the bell on the right and repeat the getup. Option 1 is usually used when going heavy, option 2 for when you're lifting light, option 3 for moderate weight.

GOOD MORNINGS

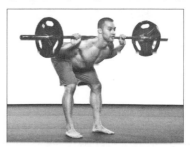

1 Place a bar in a squat rack or squat stand high enough that you can easily back up under the bar. Back up under the bar and place it across your shoulder blades, keeping your elbows down and back. Stand up to lift the bar off the hooks; walk out a few steps. **2** Push your hips back and slightly bend your knees until your back is almost parallel to the floor. **3** Squeeze and stand back up, driving your hips forward.

DEADLIFTS

Conventional Barbell Deadlift

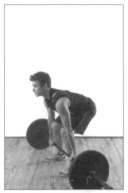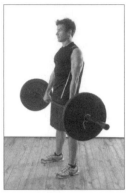

1 Stand with your feet hip-width apart. Place the bar so it's over your feet where your shoelaces would be. Push your hips back and bend your knees; keep your chest up but keep your head in line with the rest of your spine. Your back should be flat not rounded or arched. Hold the bar with one palm facing backward and the other palm facing forward. The thumbs on each hand should be on the same side of the bar as the rest of that hand (i.e., a "false" grip). **2** Drive through your heels, push your hips forward and drag the bar up your shins. As it passes your knees, straighten them. Squeeze your glutes and abs tight and stand up tall. Don't lean back. **3** To lower the bar to the floor, push your hips back and let the bar travel in a straight line, keeping it close to your thighs. As it passes your knees, bend them and sit back and down until the bar reaches the floor.

Barbell Romanian Deadlift

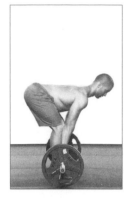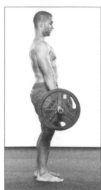

Performed like the conventional deadlift, except here your knees barely bend as your hips go straight back.

Band Sumo Deadlift

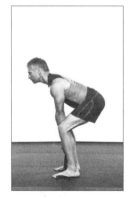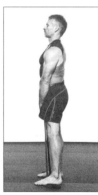

1 Stand on the band with your feet at least shoulder-width apart. Keep slack in the band between your feet; you don't need tension there. **2** Grasp the band with both hands, push your hips back and bend your knees. **3** Straighten your knees and extend your hips. Stand up tall just as though you were using a barbell.

Band Romanian Deadlift

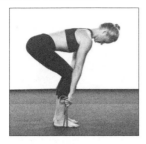

For this one, set up the same as the band sumo deadlift but, instead of bending your knees, focus on pushing your hips back (as with the barbell Romanian deadlift).

Kettlebell Sumo Romanian Deadlift

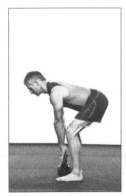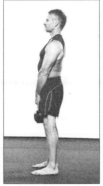

1 Straddle the kettlebell with a shoulder-width stance. **2** Push your hips way back, bend your knees a little, then grab the handle. Keep your chest lifted and your lower back arched. **3** Squeeze your abs, push your hips forward, straighten your knees and stand up tall with the bell between your legs; keep your hamstrings, glutes and abs tight.

1-Leg Kettlebell Deadlift

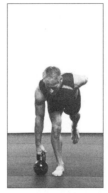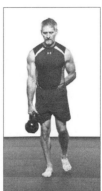

1 Stand with your feet together and the kettlebell just outside your right toes. Push your hips back and down and grab the handle with your right hand. Keep your chest up and out. Lift your left foot off the ground and straighten it behind you. There should be a straight line between the back of your head and the heel of your foot. Keep your abs tight and your hips locked to prevent your body from rotating; your hips and shoulders must remain parallel to the floor. **2–4** Drive through your right heel, leading with your shoulders, and push your hips forward. Keep your weight on the back part of your right foot. As you stand, straighten your right knee, extend your hips, and let your left leg move as a unit with the rest of your body. Return the bell to the floor by pushing your hips back and down in the exact reverse motion of how you stood up.

Double-Bell Kettlebell Deadlift

You can perform this using 2 bells. Just place the second bell by the outside of the other foot. You should go heavier with 2 bells.

Contra-Lateral Kettlebell Deadlift

For an extra challenge and more core activation, hold the bell with the hand opposite the working leg (so if you're working your right leg, hold the bell in your left hand).

1-Leg Romanian Deadlift

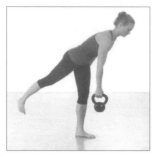

1 Very similar to the 1-Leg Kettlebell Deadlift (page 93), this version uses the back more. You basically fold through the hip with very little knee bend to lift the bell. This is a great exercise for the lower back.

Rotational 1-Leg Straight-Leg Deadlift

1 Perform the 1-Leg Deadlift with the bell in your right hand, keeping your knee as straight as possible but allowing a slight bend. **2** As you push your hips and foot back, reach across to your left and try to place the ball of the bell on the floor. Make sure your lower back stays flat throughout the movement.

CLEANS

Barbell Clean

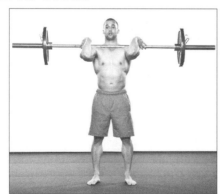

This fast, explosive movement relies on extension of the ankles, knees and hips to bring the bar up, and a quick drop under the bar to catch it in your fingers across your collar bone. This lift is somewhat technical. To become truly proficient, you need to see a certified Olympic lifting coach.

1 Start with the bar on the floor and your feet about shoulder-width apart and pointed forward. **2** Keeping your arms straight, drop your hips into a squat. Let your elbows point along the bar, not back. **3** Rapidly drive through your hips and knees and explode up. As the bar starts to pass your knees, shrug your shoulders hard. Pull hard with your arms, allowing your elbows to bend and point to your sides. The bar must stay against your thighs as it continues to travel upward. **4** As your hips and knees reach full extension, jump off the floor, extending through your ankles. When your ankles, hips and knees are fully extended, quickly pull yourself under the bar and into a deep squat. It's like someone kicked your legs out from under you. While you're pulling yourself under the bar, rotate your elbows up so that they're in front of your shoulders, your fingertips are on your collar bones, and the bar is across your fingertips. **5** Stand up.

Barbell Power Clean

This is the same as the barbell clean but you only drop into a partial squat.

Barbell Clean & Press

1 Do a barbell clean followed by a barbell overhead press (page 84).

Kettlebell Dead Clean

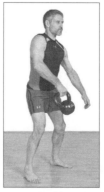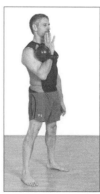

1 Stand with your feet about shoulder-width apart and the bell on the floor between your feet, angling the handle back toward your left foot. With your right arm hanging straight and your torso upright, squat down and grab the handle so that the webbing between your thumb and forefinger faces your left foot. Look out, not down.   **2** Explode through your quads and hips like you're trying to jump straight up. As your legs straighten, keep your arm relaxed; the momentum from the upward hip movement will cause the bell to rise up. As it does, shrug your shoulder a little, with your elbow coming up to about chest height.   **3** Now quickly drop your elbow into your ribs and let your forearm and hand come up, shoving your hand through the handle. Keep your thumb pointing toward your body and your wrist straight. The bell should rest on the back of your forearm and its handle should rest across the palm of your hand, diagonally from the base of your pinky to between your thumb and forefinger. You should now be in rack position.

To return the bell to the floor, bump your forearm slightly away from your body or tip your fingers toward the floor. Keeping the thumb side of your hand toward your body, bend your wrist and let the bell fall off the back of your forearm and into the crook of your fingers. Bend your legs to absorb the force. Keep your arm relaxed but maintain enough tension to hold onto the bell. Squat to place the bell on the floor with a straight elbow.

Double Kettlebell Dead Clean

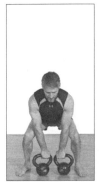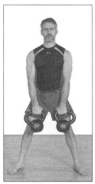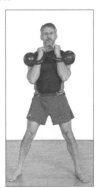

For this version, start with 2 bells on the floor between your feet.

2-Step Alternating Kettlebell Clean

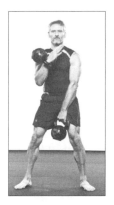

You'll need a pair of bells of the same size and weight.

1 Stand tall and hold a bell in each hand between your legs.   **2** Bend your knees and explode up. Your shoulder should naturally rise a little, followed by your arm and the bell. As your hips finish their upward movement, the bell should move straight up in front of your body. Keep your thumb turned toward you, quickly drop your elbow and drive your hand through the handle. You now have one bell in rack and one in hang position.   **3–4** Dump the racked bell back to hang position, then clean the other bell.

1-Step Alternating Clean

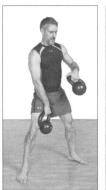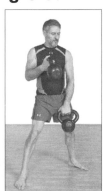

For this version, stand tall and hold a bell in each hand between your legs. Rack one bell and keep the other in hang position.

1 Dip your knees and hips and then explode up and clean the lower bell. As the lower bell begins to rise, the upper bell begins to fall. **2** As you finish the clean, bend your knees into a quarter squat to absorb the fall of the upper bell, then drive up again and switch the bells. Focus on the bell going up; the one going down will take care of itself. Your leg movements should be continuous.

SQUATS

Bodyweight Squat

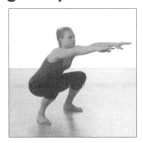

1 Stand with your feet slightly more than shoulder-width apart and feet turned out a little. **2** Squat down slowly and deliberately, keeping your torso upright as much as possible. At the same time drive your knees out so they remain pointed in the same direction as your toes. Go as deep as you can without allowing your torso to fold over or your tailbone to tuck under. Don't let your knees go forward past your toes. **3** Drive through your heels and stand, making sure the abs remain tight, and return to start position.

Goblet Squat

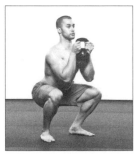

Hold a dumbbell or kettlebell chest high. If you're holding a dumbbell, it should hang vertically with you holding the top bell. With a kettlebell, hold the sides

of the handles and keep your elbows in. Don't let your elbows straighten as you squat.

Racked Squat

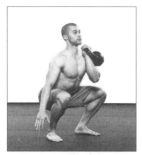

Clean a kettlebell and hold it in rack position. When squatting, keep your elbow in and down—your body moves away from the elbow, the elbow doesn't move. If you find the kettlebell is falling off your arm, you're probably folding at the waist. Stay tall and tight and try not to use the other hand to keep the bell in place. This can also be done with 2 bells.

Barbell Front Squat

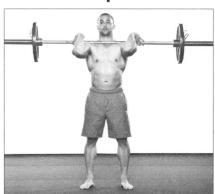

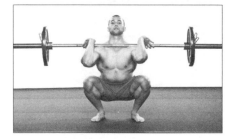

1 Clean the barbell (see page 94) or use a squat rack/ stand. **2** Keep your elbows up and shoulders packed down as you perform the squat. If your upper body pitches forward, you'll drop the bar.

Barbell Back Squat

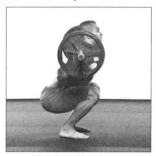

Use a squat rack or squat stand. To get really good at the back squat, you should find a coach to give you the in-depth instruction this lift requires.

1 Step backward and position the bar across your shoulder blades. Stick out your chest and try to bend the bar across your back. Keep your traps and lats tight. **2** Pull your hips back and down but keep your upper body inclined forward at the hips. This keeps your center of gravity over the midportion of your feet. The depth of your squat depends on your flexibility. You should try to get your thighs parallel to your hips or lower, however don't allow your lower back to round. **3** Drive through your heels and keep your entire midsection tight, not just your belly. Create a belt around your body by breathing into your entire lower back and sides as well as your abs.

Barbell Overhead Squat

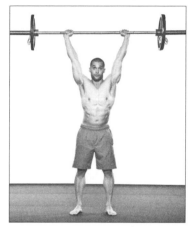

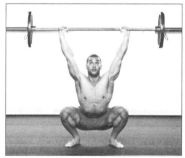

Practice this movement with a broomstick or PVC pipe and make sure you can do it properly before loading up with weight. If your shoulders aren't flexible enough to have your arms vertical overhead or you arch your back when pressing, you should stick to lighter weights and use kettlebells or dumbbells instead. You should also spend some time stretching your lats.

1 Press a barbell overhead and keep it there (see barbell press on page 84). **2** With your arms overhead and elbows locked out, stay tight and squat down as far as you can without your arms coming forward or your torso pitching forward. If you have restricted range of motion anywhere, this exercise will show you where.

Band Squat

With bands you can squat while standing on or in the band; attach the band to a fixed point and face away from it, face it or turn sideways to it. Each variation hits the core, hips and quads differently but you're still doing the same basic movement as a bodyweight squat: hips down and back, weight on the heels, knees pushed out.

Attached Band Squat—Facing

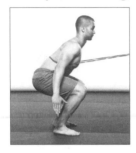

Attach a band to a stable object. Step into the band facing the attachment, positioning the band around your waist. Lean away from the attachment point from your ankles, keeping your knees, hips and back straight before you perform the squat.

Attached Band Squat—Facing Away

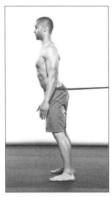

This can also be done facing away from the attachment. You should lean forward a little to keep the band from pulling you backward.

Attached Band Squat—Sideways

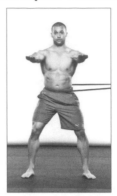

For an intense obliques workout, squat perpendicular (sideways) to the band. Keep your abs and legs centered, avoiding a weight shift away from the post.

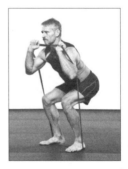

Unattached Band Squat

Stand inside a band with it looped under the middle of each foot; your feet are about shoulder-width apart. Grab the band on either side with your palms facing up and stretch it so it goes across your shoulders.

Hindu Squat

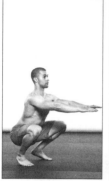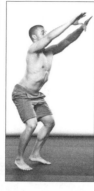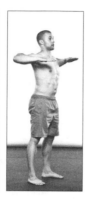

This is a deep knee bend done with arm movement in a circular, fluid, non-stop motion. If you have knee problems, stick to standard bodyweight squats, or, if your knees start to feel off in a bad way, back off the reps and speed or switch to bodyweight squats.

1 Start with your feet about hip-width apart (a slightly narrower base than a regular squat) and your toes pointed as close to straight ahead as possible. **2-3** With your arms by your sides, squat down onto the balls of your feet. Let your arms move behind you on the way down. When you reach the bottom, bring your arms forward and up to shoulder height as you stand up. At the top, your elbows should bend and your forearms should come in. Your torso should remain vertical throughout the movement.

Start slowly and learn the movement, and gradually increase the reps and speed.

Box Squat

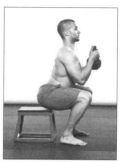

The box squat movement is the same as a goblet squat or barbell front squat—the difference is the box. Done correctly, this squat will clean up your squat pattern, activate your core and make you much stronger when doing other types of squats. If you have a lot of issues with squats, do the box squat with very light weight or none at all.

You'll need a box or an aerobics step with risers. The height of the box is determined by your flexibility level. It should be set to the point where your form breaks down. If you tend to tip forward when you go too deep, the step should be just at that point. If you go very deep and your tailbone tips under, the box or step should be set to the point just before the tip occurs.

If you use a box, stand with your legs to either side of a corner. If you're using a step, position your feet about 6 inches away from it. In both cases your feet are the same as with any other squat.

1 As you squat, push your hips back and down and try to find the box with your butt. This is a slow, controlled descent. Your butt should literally sit on the box for a 1 count before standing back up. I usually recommend a 3-count down, a 1-count hold and a 2-count back up. You should feel this is your abs, as well as your hips, glutes and quads.

Thruster

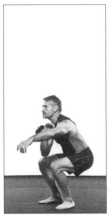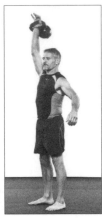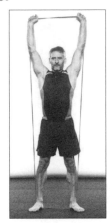

This is a very dynamic, non-stop squat and press that's very demanding to both your cardiovascular system and muscles. Make sure you can squat and press well. Don't go heavy until you figure out the flow. The thruster can be done with a barbell in rack position, 1 or 2 kettlebells in rack or 1 or 2 dumbbells held at the shoulders.

1 With your weight of choice in the proper position, squat down quickly. **2** As soon as you hit bottom, explode up and drive your arms straight up overhead. Your arms should be locked out at the same time your lower body movement is complete. **3** As soon as you hit lockout, quickly drop back into a squat. Your hands return to their start position while you're dropping down.

Band Thruster

For the band version, step inside the band with your feet shoulder-width apart and the band under the middle of each foot. With your palms face up, grab the band in each hand slightly wider than your shoulders and raise your hands to shoulder height. Squat deeply and explode up while keeping your feet on the ground. Reverse your movement by bringing the band back to shoulder height as you squat back down. To make this harder, create slack between the feet.

WINDMILLS

Kettlebell Low Windmill

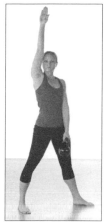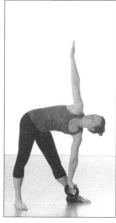

This can also be done with a dumbbell.

1 Stand with your feet about shoulder-width apart. Place a bell on the floor next to the instep of your left foot. Rotate your left hip so that the foot and knee point about 45 degrees to the left. Your right foot can either point straight ahead or also to the left. Hold your right arm straight up so that your hand is over your shoulder and your elbow is locked; try to keep it vertical throughout the movement. **2** Keeping your chest lifted and your spine straight, push your hips hard to the right and fold through the hips. Make sure your hip goes to the side, not to the rear, to prevent upper body rotation. Let your left arm slide down the inside of your leg until you can grasp the bell's handle in your left hand. Although your right arm should remain vertical the whole time, let it rotate a little as you go down, moving your body around your shoulder joint. Your knees should be straight or close to it; try to keep your right knee straight even if you have to bend your left knee a little. Keep your weight centered over your right leg. **3** Holding onto the bell with your left hand, stand up by reversing the hip movement. You should feel this in your obliques, hamstrings and glutes.

Kettlebell Overhead Windmill

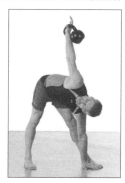

For this version, get the bell overhead by doing a clean and press or a snatch with your right arm. Keeping an eye on the bell and your shoulder in its socket at all times, push your hips hard to the right and let your left arm slide down the inside of your left leg, going as deeply as you can.

Kettlebell Double Windmill

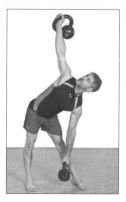

This version combines the low and overhead windmills.

ROWS

Barbell Bent Row

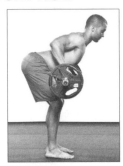

Load a barbell appropriately, not too heavy. Throughout this entire exercise, your body shouldn't change position. There's a tendency to jerk the bar or lift the torso when pulling. That means your core isn't strong enough to handle the load, so go lighter.

1 Stand with your feet about hip-width apart, toes pointed forward, and hold the barbell in both hands.   **2** Push your hips back and bend your knees a little (this is the same position as a Romanian deadlift or good morning).   **3** Keeping your chest out and initiating with your shoulder blades, pull the bar to your solar plexus.   **4** Slowly lower the bar to the start position.

There are quite a few variations of this exercise: You can change the back angle, where the bar is pulled to, whether the elbows point back or to the sides and whether the palms are face up or face down.

T-Bar Row

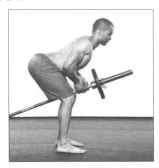

Take a free barbell and place one end in a corner or a Landmine, or use a machine specifically for this exercise, which will usually have handles. Load the other end of the bar with weight.

1 Stand over the bar with your feet behind the plates (closer to the wall). If you're using a machine, stand on the foot plates.   **2** Bend forward from your hips and grab the bar just behind the plates with both hands (or the handles if you're using a machine). Your arms should be straight.   **3** Keep your back position and pull the bar up with your arms.   **4** Slowly lower it to the floor, letting your arms straighten out.

Kettlebell/Dumbbell Row

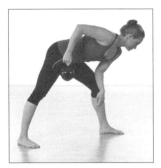

1 Place your left foot forward and your right foot back, with your feet about hip-width apart or slightly wider. Place the bell in line with your shoulder and the toes of your left foot, with the handle parallel to the foot. Keep your back flat. Place your left forearm across your left thigh, just above your knee. With your right hand, grab the bell's handle and tip it so it rests on its back bottom edge.   **2** Using your back muscles and retracting your shoulder blade, squeeze everything tight and pull the bell to your hip. Don't let your shoulders or hips turn, or let your torso move up and down. Keep your whole body locked in place.   **3** Slowly return the bell to its start position on the floor.

1-Arm 1-Leg Underhand-Grip Dumbbell Row

You'll need a dumbbell and a bench or squat rack to hold.

1 Raise one leg off the floor behind you and place the opposite hand on the bench for support. Hold the dumbbell in your free hand with an underhand grip (palm facing forward), arm hanging straight down.   **2** Pull the dumbbell to your side. Keep your torso parallel to the floor and your hips level. Don't allow your hips or torso to rotate.   **3** Slowly lower the bell.

Standing Band Row

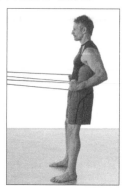

You can do this with both arms working together or alternating. Mix it up.

1 Attach the band(s) to a sturdy post, a squat rack or even a tree, then step about 2 feet away from the attachment site.   **2** Facing the attachment, use your lats to pull the bands back to your hips in a rowing motion.

1-Arm Standing Band Row

From Standing Band Row, take a staggered stance and hold the band with one hand. Contracting your core so you don't rotate or get pulled off balance by the band,

pull the band to your bottom ribs. Your elbow should just pass 90 degrees.

Rotational Band Pull

This is an explosive movement; use a heavier band. From 1-Arm Standing Band Row, rotate your hips to the same side as you pull the band to your side. This lets the abs help, dynamically working the obliques. Rotate your hips back to the front as you extend your arm.

Tall Kneeling Band Row

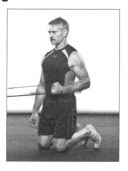

You may want a yoga mat or something similar to pad your knees. Kneel down with both knees on the floor so that they're not touching each other. Your thighs should be vertical front and side. Squeeze your glutes and keep your hips under you as you row. You should feel your abs and glutes kick in hard to keep you from falling over.

Half Kneeling Band Row

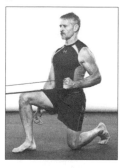

Place one knee on the floor and step the other foot in front of you, bending the knee 90 degrees. The front shin and back thigh are vertical; you should be on the ball of the rear foot. Stay tight and squeeze your glutes, keeping your hips under you. Pull from the down-side arm.

Seated Pulley Row

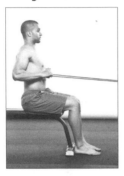

Don't let the torso collapse, bend, twist or lean back.

1 Sit on a bench with your feet flat on the floor, torso forward. Stay tall. Your arms should be extended about even with your upper chest.   **2** Grab the handle with your arms straight and no slack in the cable.   **3** Initiating the pull from your shoulder blades, continue to pull back until your forearms are touching your lower ribs. Your upper arms will be slightly off vertical. Don't pull too far back. If you feel it in the front of your shoulders, you're bringing your elbows too far back.   **4** Slowly extend your arms.

Bodyweight Row

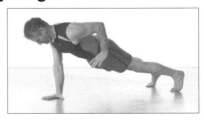

1 Assume a high plank and pull one hand back to your hip, utilizing your lats to retract your shoulder blade. Make sure you keep your hips and abs tight—there should be no rotation in the hips or waist.   **2** Lower your hand and repeat on the other side.

Kettlebell Renegade Row

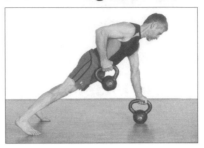

This can also be done with dumbbells.

1 Position the bells so that the handles are shoulder-width apart and parallel to your body. Place the hip of each hand (at the base of the little finger) on a handle and wrap your fingers around it; this grip will help keep your wrists straight. Assume a high plank/push-up position and lock out your hips.   **2** Keeping everything tight, slowly pull one bell up to your hip. *Note:* Any movement of the supporting arm or hand can make you fall. Avoid letting your hips come up or rotating your hips or torso.   **3** Slowly lower the bell back to the start position, shift your weight to lift the other bell and repeat on the other side.

Modification: If you can't prevent your hips from coming up or your hips/torso from rotating, move your feet farther apart. If you still can't do it, use lighter bells or do it without bell (see Chest Touch below).

Chest Touch

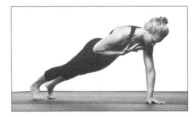

1 Start in a high plank position and lock everything tight, keeping your hips extended.   **2** Quickly touch one hand to your chest and bring it back to the floor.

Repeat with the other arm. Move quickly but try to keep your hips from moving side to side or up and down.

WEIGHTED WALKS

Farmer's Walk

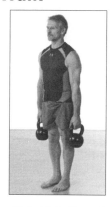

This can be done with kettlebells or dumbbells

1 Pick up 2 heavy bells. Stand tall, keep your shoulders in their sockets and walk. Make sure not to lean forward—keep your chest up and shoulders back at all times.

Waiter's Walk

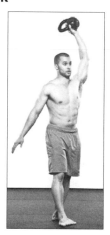

Hold 1 or 2 bells overhead and walk. With kettlebells you can either hold the handle in your palm and the bell on the outside of your forearm, or you can hold the ball portion of the bell in your palm with your palm facing up. Keep your elbows locked and walk. If you have shoulder mobility issues, don't do doubles.

Offset Walk

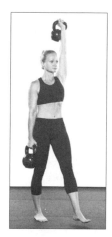

This combines the farmer's walk and the waiter's walk. Hold one bell down and a lighter one overhead and walk for the specified time or distance before switching.

LAT PULL-DOWN

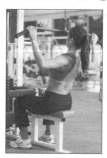

Sit on a bench facing the machine, knees under the supports.

1 Hold the bar so your hands are slightly wider than your shoulders but not too wide. Maintain a flat back and tall spine. **2** Lean back slightly from your hips and, initiating with your back, pull the bar to your chest. Pinch your shoulder blades together to make sure your lats—not your biceps—are doing the work. Keep your shoulder blades down.

UPRIGHT ROWS

Barbell Upright Row

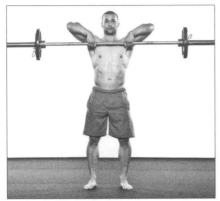

1 Stand tall holding a barbell in front of you with straight arms and both palms facing back. Your hands should be in front of your thighs. Note that keeping both hands at the center of the bar can make a shoulder impingement worse. **2** Stay tight and pull the bar straight up until the bar is shoulder height. Your elbows should be higher than your hands and flared to the sides. **3** Lower the bar with control to the start position.

SHRUGS

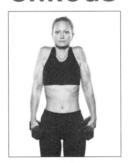

This can be done with a trap bar or 1 or 2 kettlebells/ dumbbells.

1 Stand with your feet hip-width apart and hold the weights with your arm(s) hanging straight down alongside your thigh(s). If you're using a trap bar, your arms will be wider. **2** Shrug your shoulders hard, hold and then slowly release.

DELTOID RAISES

Lateral Raise

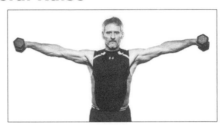

This exercise works primarily the lateral aspect of the deltoids.

1 Hold a dumbbell in each hand in front of your thighs with your palms facing each other. Keeping a neutral spine, bend slightly at your hips and knees. Don't round your back. **2** Keeping the movement slow and controlled, raise your arms directly up to the sides, with your elbows slightly bent throughout the movement. At the top, your arms should be parallel to the floor, elbows at the same level as the wrists or a little higher.

Rear Lateral Raise

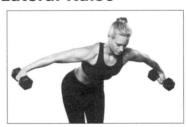

This works the posterior deltoids and is almost the reverse of the flye movement.

1 Hold a dumbbell in each hand in front of your thighs with your palms facing each other. Keeping a neutral spine, fold through your hips and slightly bend your knees. Your torso should almost be parallel to the floor. The bells should now be hanging in front of your knees. **2** With control, raise the bells up to the sides, keeping your elbows bent around 10 degrees, even with or slightly higher than your wrists. Keep the pinkie side of your hand a little higher than the thumb side.

Cable Lateral Raise

You'll need a cable system that has 2 sides so you can stand between them. You can substitute 2 bands if you have attachment points that are about 6–8 feet apart that you can stand between. Set the cables or bands low. Stand tall and hold one handle in each hand, arms crossed in front in the low position. Don't lean forward as that changes which portions of the deltoids work.

1 Raise your arms to the sides until they're shoulder height. Elbows are slightly bent throughout the movement.   **2** Slowly lower your arms in front of you until they cross again.

Cable Crossover

This is basically the reverse of the cable lateral raise.

1 Stand between 2 cables set in the high position, with your arms about shoulder height and your elbows slightly bent and pointed back. Bend forward a little from your knees and hips.   **2** Keeping your elbows slightly bent, squeeze your pecs and bring your hands down in front of you. Pretend you're hugging a tree.

Front Raise

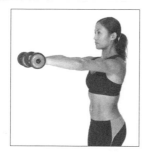

1 Stand with a dumbbell in each hand, arms straight down and palms facing the rear.   **2** With control, raise both arms in an arc to the front and up until your hands are a little higher than your shoulders. Don't try to force the range of motion. Only raise as high as you can without arching your back or otherwise cheating.

PRESS-DOWNS

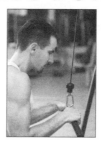

This requires a machine, either cables or a weight stack system.

1 Attach a pull-down bar to the cable. Stand facing the machine with the bar about chest height. Grab the bar with an overhead grip (palms facing floor). Your forearms should be touching your upper body.   **2** Squeeze your whole body and push the bar downward in an arc by straightening your elbows while they stay pinned to your sides.

CURLS

Barbell Curl

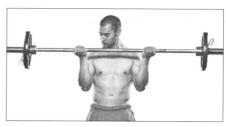

1 Hold a barbell in front of your thighs, palms facing forward, arms straight, elbows against your sides.   **2** Squeeze your core, bend your elbows and bring your hands and the bar up toward your chest/ shoulders while keeping your elbows against your sides. Don't jerk or use momentum. Slow, controlled movement will give you the best results.   **3** With control, lower the bar to the start position. Don't allow your torso to bend as the bar goes down.

EZ-Bar Curl

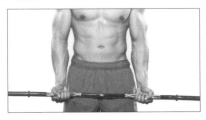

When using an EZ-bar instead of a barbell, hold the bar so that your palms face forward and toward your center line.

Band Curl

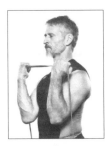

For this version, stand inside a band with your palms facing forward.

Seated Dumbbell Curl

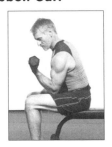

Sit on a bench and place your elbow on your thigh, with the forearm along the thigh.

Incline Dumbbell Curl

Using a pair of dumbbells, lie face up on an incline bench.

Dumbbell Hammer Curl

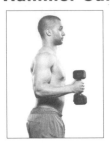

1 Hold a dumbbell in each hand with your arms straight alongside your thighs, palms facing inward. **2** With control, bring your hands up toward each shoulder, keeping your elbows against your sides. The thumb side of your hand remains up throughout the entire movement.

Band Hammer Curl

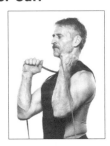

Stand inside a band so it's under the middle portion of each foot. Hold one end of the band in each hand, arms straight down and palms facing each other.

Concentration Curl

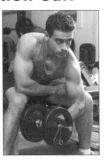

1 Sit on a bench with your feet apart and hold a dumbbell in one hand. Place your elbow on your inner thigh about midway. **2** Straighten your elbow until your arm is fully extended, then bend your elbow to bring the dumbbell back up.

Dumbbell Curl with Alternating Lunge

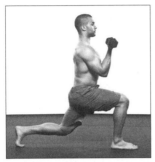

1 Stand with a dumbbell in each hand. **2** As you step into a forward lunge (page 113), curl the bells to shoulder height. **3** Return to standing, letting your arms return to the start position.

Alternate legs with each rep.

Alternating Curl & Lunge

You may also curl one side as you step out, return to standing, then step out with the other foot and curl that side.

Forearm Curl

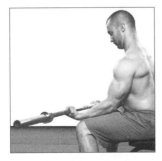

1 Sit on a bench with either a barbell or 1 or 2 dumbbells in your hands, palms face up. Place your forearms on your thighs, which should be parallel to the floor. If they're not, place a weight plate under each foot to get your thighs parallel. You can either keep the backs of your hands on your thighs or move your forearms so that your wrists hang in front of your knees, increasing

the range of motion and difficulty. **2** Keeping your forearms on your thighs, bend your wrists to bring the weights toward your body. **3** Slowly reverse the movement until your palms are face up again (hands on thighs) or facing forward in front of your knees.

Reverse Curl

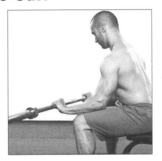

1 Sit on a bench with either a barbell or 1 or 2 dumbbells in your hands, palms face down and hanging in front of your knees. **2** Bend your wrists backward to bring the weights closer to your torso.

Wrist Roller

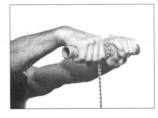

You'll need a 2-foot-long stick, a ⅜"- to ½"-rope that's 5 feet long, a barbell plate and a 3" stick or metal rod. Tie the rope to the middle of the long stick; you'll probably have to use duct tape to keep it from slipping around. Thread the other end of the rope through the plate and tie it to the short stick or rod.

1 Stand tall and extend your arms in front of you, holding one end of the long stick in each hand, elbows straight and palms facing the floor at shoulder height. **2** Grip the stick tightly with one hand and curl that wrist back. At the same time, allow the stick to rotate through the other hand. When you've reached the end range of motion of the first wrist, grip the stick more tightly with the second hand and relax the grip of the first hand.   **3** Flex the wrist of the second hand and at the same time extend the other wrist but allow the stick to move through the first hand.   **4** When you've hit end range of motion of the second hand, grab the stick firmly with the first hand, relax the grip of the second hand, pull the first wrist back toward you and push the second wrist forward.

Continue until the rope is wound up all the way. When done, reverse the movement so that you're gripping while extending the wrist and relaxing the other hand and flexing it. Continue until the rope is unwound.

TRICEPS

Triceps Kickback

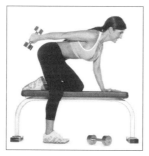

1 Kneel on a bench with one knee and place the other foot flat on the floor slightly behind the elevated knee. Place the hand on the same side as the elevated knee on the bench to support your upper body. Your back should be flat. Hold a light dumbbell in your free hand so that the elbow is bent 90 degrees with the forearm hanging down vertically. Your upper arm should be parallel to your back.   **2** Without moving your upper arm or changing your elbow position, lift the dumbbell behind you until your arm is straight and parallel to your back, which should be parallel to the floor.   **3** Bend your elbow and return your forearm to the start position.

Triceps Extension

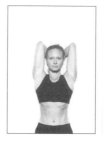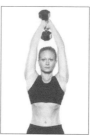

Choose a weight that'll let you bend your elbows completely. This can also be done with 1 arm at a time.

1 Stand or sit with a tall, neutral spine. Hold a dumbbell or kettlebell in both hands over your head.   **2** Bend your elbows until the weight is behind your head.   **3** Extend your arms overhead until your elbows are locked out.

Band Triceps Extension

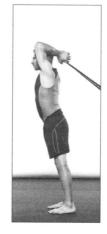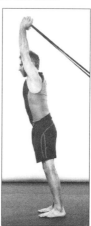

This can be done with 1 or 2 hands.

1 Attach a band to something sturdy. Face away from the attachment in a staggered stance (easier) or even stance (more core). Bend your elbow so that it's above and behind your head, and grab the band.   **2** Leaning forward slightly, straighten your elbow. Your arm should be in a straight line with your back—don't pull the band around your ears. Don't let the band pull you backward or jerk you out of position, and try not to bend at the waist.   **3** Slowly bend your elbow back.

Band Bent-Over Triceps Extension

This can be done with 1 heavy band using both arms or 2 lighter bands, one in each hand. It's like the regular band triceps extension (page 110), except here you push your hips back with knees slightly bent so that your torso is close to parallel to the floor.

Dumbbell Pullover

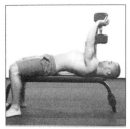

Choose a weight that'll let you bend your elbows completely.

1 Lie on a bench with your feet on the floor and hold a dumbbell with both hands over your sternum, arms straight but elbows slightly bent. If your feet don't reach the floor, place some weight plates under your feet. **2** Keeping your lower back pressed into the bench, slowly lower the dumbbell over your head until your arms are parallel to the floor. Range of motion will depend on your shoulder mobility—stop when you feel the stretch in your shoulders or chest. **3** Slowly bring your arms back to vertical.

Barbell French Press

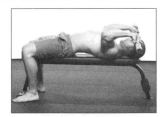

This triceps extension exercise is also known as the "Skullcrusher."

1 Lie face up on a bench and have a spotter hand you a barbell. Keep your arms vertical and your palms facing forward. **2** Bend your elbows until the bar almost

touches your forehead. **3** Extend your elbows until your arms are vertical again.

Dumbbell French Press

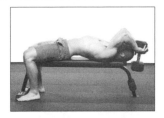

This can also be done with dumbbells, with either one dumbbell in each hand or one dumbbell in both hands. When doing it with one dumbbell in both hands, the dumbbell goes behind your head.

Dip

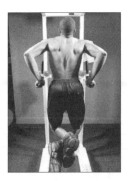

You'll need a dip station, gymnastics rigs or some other way to lift your body off the ground by pushing up with your arms. Note that versions where you have your hands on a bench or chair behind you and your legs out in front can put a lot of stress on the shoulders.

1 Get into the dip station and hold the pads. Leaning forward a little is okay, but leaning too far forward can aggravate shoulder issues. **2** Squeeze tight and lower yourself until you feel a slight stretch in your shoulders or chest. **3** Push your body back up.

Triple Crush

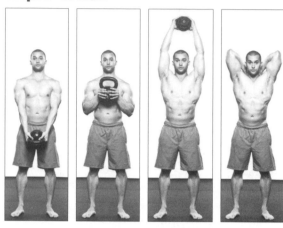

This hits the biceps, triceps and core and can be done with a kettlebell or dumbbell. The weight you use will be dictated by how strong your triceps are.

1 Stand with your feet hip-width apart. Hold a bell in front of your pelvis and keep your elbows as straight as possible. Don't lean forward.   **2** Keeping your elbows tight against your body, bend them and bring the bell to your chest.   **3** Press the bell directly overhead. If you feel your back arch excessively, you should avoid this move until you're more flexible. Try not to lean forward.   **4** With the bell overhead, bend your elbows to bring the bell behind your head. Try to completely bend your elbows and keep them pointed forward.   **5** Squeeze your body and straighten your elbows, bringing the bell back to overhead position.   **6** Pull the bell back so it's in front of your chest.   **7** Bend your elbows to bring the bell back to the start position.

CALF RAISES
Standing Calf Raise

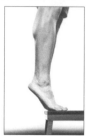

If these are easy, add weight by wearing a weight vest. You won't really be able to hold a weight because you'll need your hands for balance.

1 Stand on the edge of a step or anything that'll let your heels hang off of it. You may want to position yourself so you have something to hold onto with your hands.   **2** Slowly lower your heels as far as possible.   **3** Slowly lift your heels as high as possible.

Standing Calf Raise–Weighted

If standard calf raises are easy, add weight by wearing a weight vest. You won't really be able to hold a weight because you'll need your hands for balance. Your other option is to use a dedicated machine that will allow you to add weight; stand with the pads on your shoulders. Hold the top position briefly to work your body harder.

Seated Calf Raise

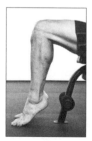

1 Sit on the edge of bench with your feet flat on the floor.   **2** Raise your heels as high as possible.

Seated Calf Raise–Weighted

Place a weight across your thighs for increased difficulty.

1-Leg Calf Raise

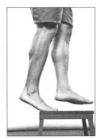

Perform a calf raise while standing on one leg.

LUNGES

Static Lunge

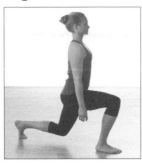

This, also known as a split squat, is a very important exercise. If you wobble or lose your alignment, you're not ready for more advanced lunge variations. If you feel this in either knee, you're pushing with your toes. The front leg does most of the work, the back foot mostly balances. Pay attention to your torso angle, hips, glutes and front knee.

1 Step one foot out a little farther than your natural step and raise your back heel. Your back heel should be lifted throughout the lunge.   **2** Bend your knees until they're 90 degrees. Your front thigh should be parallel to the floor and your front shin should be vertical.   **3** With an upright torso and hips under you, squeeze your abs, glutes and quads and drive off your front heel and stand

tall. Your front knee will not lock out but your back knee will.

Switch sides.

Forward Lunge

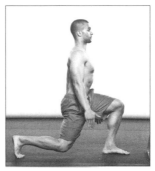

Make sure you can do a static lunge with minimal problems before trying this.

1 Stand with your feet hip-width apart.   **2** Leading with your heel, step forward with one leg; the distance should be a little more than your normal stride length. Sink your hips straight down into a lunge.   **3** Driving through your front heel, come up tall and step your lead foot back to the start position. For beginners, the return to start is a 2-step move; for intermediate to advanced, it's one.

Lunge to Step-Up

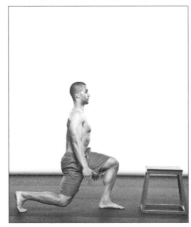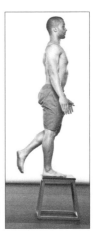

This advanced lunge variation requires good flexibility, mobility and stability. Make sure you can do a static lunge with minimal problems before trying this. You'll need a sturdy box or aerobics step. Set it to the same height as the top of your shin, the big knobby bone below the knee cap. If you have to throw your body into the stepping action or otherwise cheat, the step is too high.

1 Start in a half kneeling (lunge) position with the box or step set up a few inches in front of your lead foot. **2** Rise up out of the lunge and continue the motion by bringing the back foot completely on the box, driving through and extending the hip. Don't put the other foot on the step. **3** The foot that came up last goes back first. Place the foot flat on the floor, then step down with the other foot, placing the ball of the foot on the ground and then the knee, returning to half kneeling.

Lunge & Rotation

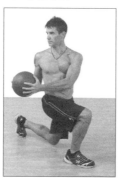

This can be done with a medicine ball, a dumbbell held by the head, or a kettlebell held by the sides of the handle.

1 Stand with your feet hip-width apart and hold a ball or bell in both hands at your chest. **2** Step your right foot forward into a lunge. **3** At the bottom of your lunge, turn your torso toward the right, keeping your hands in front of your chest. **4** Rotate back to center before standing up with feet together and repeating to the other side.

Reverse Lunge

Make sure you have the static lunge and forward lunge (page 113) down pat first.

1 Stand with your feet hip-width apart. **2** Step backward with one foot until you're in the exact same position as the top of the static lunge. **3** Staying tight, sink your hips down. Try to keep your torso upright at all times—think about someone pulling you from a rope or band wrapped around your hips. **4** Drive through your front heel to come up and step forward, bringing your feet back together.

Side Lunge

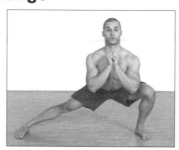

1 Stand with your feet together. **2** Step out directly to the side with one leg and sink your hips back and down. Your upper body will be inclined but keep your chest up and your hips and torso facing forward. Your other leg should be straight, with your knee in line with your middle toes. Don't let your shoulder go out past your knee. **3** Drive off the leg you stepped with and return to standing.

Dumbbell Side Lunge & Touch

Hold a dumbbell in each hand with your arms by your sides then perform a side lunge. As you get close to the floor, touch the dumbbells on the floor—one on either side of the foot.

Skater's Lunge

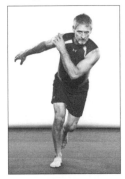

This is the movement Olympic speed skaters do. Be soft with the landings.

1 Stand with your feet together. **2** Keeping your hips back and your back straight, jump to one side, landing on one foot and letting the trailing leg swing behind the lead leg. The lead foot should be pointed almost straight ahead. Beginners can touch the trailing leg to the floor. As with all lunges and squats, make sure your knee tracks with your toes. **3** Jump to the other side so that the trailing leg now becomes the lead leg.

3-Way Lunge

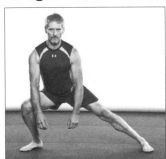

This combines the forward, side and reverse lunges.

1 Do a front lunge, return to standing and with the same foot go into a side lunge. **2** Return to standing and, still using the first foot, step into a back lunge.

After you've done all 3, switch sides.

Band Front Lunge

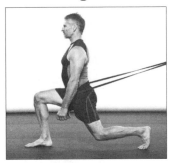

1 Attach the band to something sturdy then step inside it so it's around your hips. Move forward so that there's no slack in the band, but be careful not to put too much tension in the band or it'll pull you off balance when you stand up. **2** Step into a forward lunge. Lean forward slightly as you hit the bottom position to keep the band from pulling you backward.

Barbell Lunge–Overhead

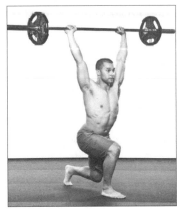

Caution: Don't do these if you have tight shoulders or shoulder problems. You must also have the flexibility to keep your torso perfectly upright. If you can't do a regular lunge, don't do it with weight overhead.

1 Clean and press a barbell. **2** With your elbows locked, step forward into a lunge. **3** Drive through your front heel to return to standing.

Barbell Lunge–Shoulder

For this version, place a bar in a squat rack or stand, then back up to it and position the bar across your shoulder blades. Keep your shoulder blades pinched together. As with the barbell overhead lunge, you must also have the flexibility to keep your torso perfectly upright. If you can't do a regular lunge, don't do this.

Rear Foot Elevated Split Squat

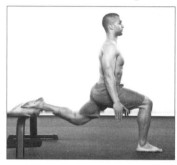

This is also known as the Bulgarian split squat.

1 Place the top of one foot on the bench, pointing the knee down; your other foot should be forward enough so that your shin is vertical when your front thigh is parallel to the floor. Straighten your front leg. Keep your torso upright throughout the exercise. **2** Bend both knees to lower your hips until your front thigh is parallel to the floor. If you feel excessive stretching through the hip flexor and quadriceps of the elevated leg, you need to stretch more; in the meantime don't go quite so deep.

Return to standing by driving with the front foot. Minimize the use of the elevated foot. It's on the bench for balance, not to help you move or stand. Keep your front foot flat on the floor throughout the entire movement.

Weighted Rear Foot Elevated Split Squat

Once you can do the unloaded movement properly, you can challenge yourself by holding a kettlebell or dumbbell chest high with both hands (the goblet position) or holding one in each hand with your arms along your sides.

CORE

Jack Knife

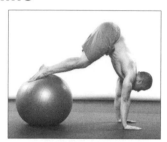

1 Place your belly on a stability ball and roll forward until your shins are on the ball and your hands are on the floor about shoulder-width apart. Keep your elbows straight and your legs straight behind you. Maintain neutral spine and don't bend at the waist throughout the movement. **2** Contract your abs and bring your knees toward your chest until your heels are close to your glutes. Your shins will move forward and the tops of your feet will contact the top of the ball. Don't let your lower back round. Hold for a breath. **3** Extend your hips back until your legs are straight.

Bird Dog

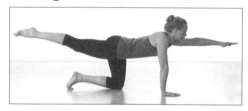

Two basic phases precede the full bird dog—once you can hold either arm out for at least 30 seconds and you can do the same with each leg with no rotation, it's time to do the full bird dog.

1 Start with your hands under your shoulders and both knees on the floor under your hips. Your thighs should be vertical from the front as well as the sides. **2** In the most basic version, lift one arm straight out in front of you at shoulder height, fingers pointing straight ahead, and hold it. Don't let your hips rotate; they and your shoulders should remain parallel to the floor. If you can hold this easily for at least 30 seconds on each side, move on to the next level. **3** For the next phase, keep both hands on the floor and lift one leg off the floor so that the leg is level with the hip and the toes point straight back. Stay tight and don't let your torso rotate. Your hips should remain parallel to the floor. **4** For the full bird dog, lift one leg and the opposite arm. As with the easier progressions, your hips and shoulders should remain parallel to the floor. There should be a straight line from your heel to your fingers. *Remember:* You're going across the body, right foot and left hand and vice versa.

Bird Dog from Plank

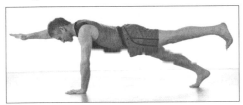

If you can do the full bird dog for at least 1 minute per side, try the full bird dog from a high plank position. This is very tough.

Forearm Plank

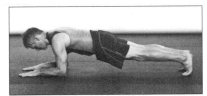

1 Place your forearms on the floor parallel to each other; align your elbows under your shoulders. You may keep your palms face down on the floor or place the outer edges of your hands/fists on the floor. Extend your legs behind you like you would for a push-up, keeping your hips in the same plane as your shoulders. Squeeze your abs, glutes, hamstrings, quads, arms—everything but your neck—and hold that position. Make sure your back is flat; don't let your back sag or your hips go high or low.

High Plank

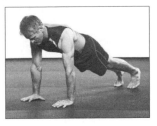

Instead of working from your forearms, assume the top position of a push-up, placing your hands on the floor in line with your shoulders.

Plank & Reach

While in plank, slowly reach forward and touch a KB/DB.

Super Plank

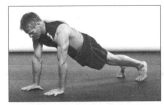

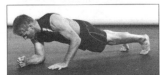

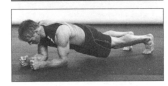

1 Start in a push-up position with your hands under your shoulders and your legs extended behind you. **2** Place one forearm on the floor so that the elbow is under the shoulder and the hand is straight out in front. **3** Now place the other forearm on the floor so that you're in a forearm plank. **4** Place one hand under the shoulder and start to straighten out that elbow. **5** As your torso starts to come up, lift the other forearm up and place that hand under the shoulder and finish straightening your elbows. You should be back in a push-up position.

Mix up the order you move the arms to keep it interesting. Don't slide your arms up and down or you'll get carpet burn. Pick up the hand and place the forearm down. It's a very distinct movement.

Side Plank

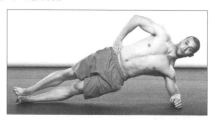

1 Lie on the floor on your side. Place your forearm on the floor so that the elbow is directly under the bottom shoulder. Stack your shoulders, hips, legs and feet.   **2** Lift your torso, hips and legs off the ground. Push your hips forward and make a straight line from the back of your head to your heels. Keep your entire body facing forward. Don't allow your torso or hips to rotate up or down. Hold, squeezing your abs and glutes hard.

Switch sides.

Side Plank with Hip Raise

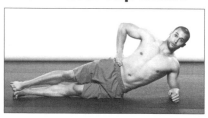

1 Assume side plank position.   **2** Stay tight and lower your hips to the floor.   **3** Lift your hips up as high as possible. As you do the up-and-down movement make sure you're still maintaining a straight back with no rotation—your body still faces forward. Also, don't let your head drop out of alignment with the rest of your spine.

Rotational Side Plank

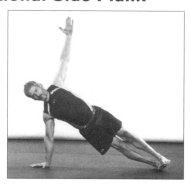

1 Start in a side plank and hold the top arm straight up.   **2** While holding the plank, rotate your torso toward the floor to reach your arm underneath you.   **3** Return to side plank, repeat, then switch sides.

Unicycle

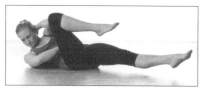

1 Lie flat on your back and place your left hand behind your head. Lift both feet about 6 inches off the floor.   **2** Contract your abs and bring your left elbow toward your hips and your right knee toward your elbow. They should meet halfway. The other leg should remain extended and about 6 inches off the floor. Don't pull on your neck with your hand!   **3** Extend your left leg and lower your torso so you're flat again.

Repeat, then switch sides, right elbow and left knee.

Waist Twist

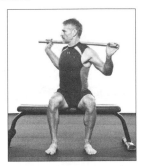

This was one of the main exercises Bruce Lee did to get his phenomenal abs. However, it can hurt your back and I don't recommend it very much. You'll need a stick or broomhandle and a chair or bench.

1 Sit tall on a bench and place the stick across your shoulders behind your neck. **2** Slowly twist from the waist as far as possible to one side and then back to the other side. Most of the movement should come from the middle and upper back, not the waist.

Sit-Up Twist

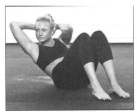

Although this is a classic move, I much prefer the unicycle (page 118) as it's much less stressful to the lower back.

1 Lie on the floor face up and place your feet flat on the floor about hip-width apart, knees bent and apart. Place your hands behind your neck. **2** Contract your abs and lift your torso off the floor. As you come up, rotate so that your right elbow approaches your left knee. **3** Lower yourself to the floor and then come back up and bring your left elbow toward your right knee. Try to keep your lower back flat as you come up.

Roman Chair Sit-Up

This is actually a supine back hyperextension into a sit-up. These are tough and may cause back problems so use caution.

1 Get into the apparatus with your face up, feet under the pads and lower back on the back support pad. Cross your arms and lay them across your chest. Bend backward as far as possible. **2** Contract your abs and sit up.

Hanging Leg Raise

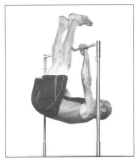

You'll need a pull-up bar. You may also want someone to keep an eye on your lower back and to stop you from swaying at the bottom. These should be done slowly with no momentum. If you feel this in your back, you're using your back (wrong) instead of your hips (right).

1 Grab a pull-up bar with your palms facing away from you. Hang with your arms straight and legs straight under you. **2** Contract your abs and use your hips to bring your knees as high as possible while keeping your legs straight. Minimize the rounding of your lower back.

Lower your legs with control. Come to a dead hang before starting the next rep.

Weighted Knee Raise

Use a vertical knee raise machine and ankle weights. Some dip stations can be used for this as well—look for forearm pads that are parallel to the floor and high enough off the ground that your legs can hang under you.

1 Get into the apparatus, with forearms on the supports, body facing outward and legs hanging under you. **2** Contract your abs and bring your knees to your chest, but don't round your lower back. **3** Slowly lower your legs using your abs and legs to resist—not your back.

Knee Raise from Pull-Up Bar

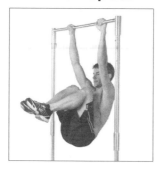

This uses a pull-up bar and, if desired, ankle weights. Hang from the pull-up bar and try to bring your knees as high as possible without rounding your back.

Pullover Crunch

1 Lie on your back with knees bent and feet flat on the floor. Hold a kettlebell on the floor behind your head tightly in both hands, with elbows bent about 90 degrees. **2** Keeping your elbows bent 90 degrees, pull the bell over your head. As it does so, sit up about halfway, pulling your elbows to your hip bones. **3** As you lie back down, bring the bell back to the floor behind your head.

Frog Kick

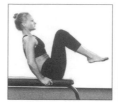 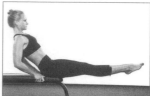

1 Sit at the end of a sturdy bench and lean back, holding the sides of the bench with both hands. Bring your knees in to your chest, but don't round your lower back. **2** Extend your knees and hips and try to get your legs parallel to the floor. **3** Contract your abs and bring your knees back in.

Glute Bridge

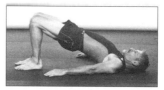

You should feel this in your butt and hamstrings. If you feel this in your lower back, you're either not firing the right muscles or you're lifting too high and arching your lower back.

1 Lie on the floor face up with knees bent and both feet flat on the floor. **2** Drive your heels into the floor and lift your hips. Keep your lower back neutral—don't arch or sag. Hold for at least 2 deep belly breaths.

Single-Leg Glute Bridge

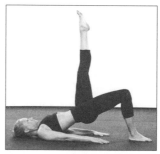

For this version, start with one leg either extended up to the ceiling or pulled toward your chest. Don't forget to switch sides.

Weighted Glute Bridge

Place a dumbbell or kettlebell just below your navel and perform the glute bridge. Some people will also use a barbell across the front of the hips.

Incline Glute Bridge

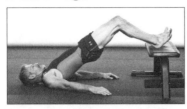

This more-challenging version starts with your feet on a bench and the rest of your body on the floor.

Leg Thrust

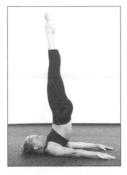

1 Lie on your back with your legs straight, then lift your feet until your hips are at a 90-degree angle to your waist; keep your feet straight over your hips. You can place your hands behind your head or by your sides. **2** Now point your toes and drive your hips up as high as you can, keeping your legs perpendicular to the floor. Your weight is on your upper back and shoulders, not your neck. **3** Lower your hips back down, then, still keeping your knees straight, lower your feet to the floor until they're about 2 inches off the floor.

Back Extension

1 Using the back extension apparatus, put your feet on the bottom plate so you're face down, the pad against the Achilles tendons on each ankle. Your hips should be just above the top of the pad; adjust as necessary. Cross your arms in front of your chest and maintain a tall, neutral spine, as if you have a board along your spine. **2** Keeping your abs tight and spine straight, exhale and slowly fold through your hips to lower your upper body. Don't go past 90 degrees of hip flexion and don't round your back! Inhale at the bottom. **3** Exhale and come back up, maintaining a tall neutral spine. Don't go beyond neutral.

Back Extension on Ball

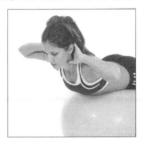

1 Place your hips on a stability ball and the bottoms of your feet against a wall. Place your hands behind your head and fold through your hips, stopping when you feel your back start to round. **2** Moving slowly and deliberately, contract your back muscles to raise your torso off the ball. Don't hyperextend your back. **3** Lower down to start position.

Pallof Press

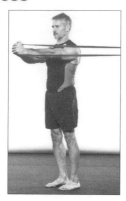

This can be performed with a band or cable.

1 Stand perpendicular to the attachment point of a medium or lighter band. Step directly to the side and hold the band in front of your chest with both hands. Your feet are hip-width apart. There should be no slack between your hands and the attachment point. **2** Keeping your hands in front of your sternum, slowly press both arms straight out. Don't lean, and don't allow your body to move, rotate or be pulled out of position by the band. Use your abs and glutes to stay in position. Hold the extended position for a 1 count then slowly bring your hands to your sternum.

Wood Chop

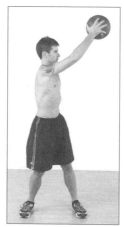

This can be done with a dumbbell, kettlebell or medicine ball.

1 Stand with your feet shoulder-width apart. Hold a medicine ball in both hands up and out to the side of the right shoulder, rotating through the upper back and a little at the hips. **2** Pull the ball down and across your body in a strong chopping movement until the bell is just outside your left knee. Your knees will be bent slightly. **3** Keeping your back flat throughout the movement, quickly reverse to return to start. You may pivot on the ball of your foot to get more power. When the bell is at the top position up to the right, pivot on the ball of your left foot with your left heel up. When you chop, plant your left heel and pivot on the ball of your right foot, raising your heel.

Ab Rollout

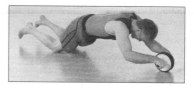

1 Kneel on the floor (with a yoga mat under your knees for padding if you wish) and hold the axle of the wheel in each hand. **2** Keeping your abs tight, push from your hips to move forward. Let your arms move ahead of you and keep your head down. To reduce stress on your lower back, keep it rounded, not flat or arched. Go out as far as you can, extending your hips if possible but not letting your thighs touch the floor.

To return to kneeling, stay tight and pull back with your hips; avoid jerking with your arms to get them back under you and keep your chin slightly tucked under.

Variation

If you can do at least 5 full ab rollouts from your knees, try starting from your feet. This is much harder—move slowly and stay tight or you'll do a faceplant. Another option is to roll out as far as you can from standing then drop to your knees, finish the rollout then reverse by pulling back to the low start position and finish by lifting your hips and pulling the rest of the way back in.

Stability Ball Rollout

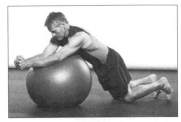

1 Place your forearms on a stability ball and your knees on the floor. **2** Keeping your back flat, roll the ball forward by moving from your hips. **3** When you can't go any farther without your back sagging or otherwise losing your alignment, squeeze your abs and glutes and return to the start position. Keep your back flat.

Side Bend

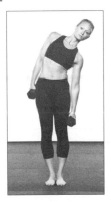

1 Hold a kettlebell or dumbbell in one hand, or hold one in each hand. Stand tall with your feet under your hips, your arms hanging straight, palms facing your thighs. **2** Bend through the last few ribs directly to the side, with no rotation of the shoulders.

If you have a weight in each hand, repeat to the other side. If not, repeat to the bell side, then switch hands.

Leaning Twist

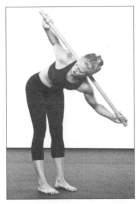

Along with waist twist (page 119), this is another of Bruce Lee's favorite ab exercises.

1 Place a stick or broomhandle on your shoulders, behind your neck. Fold forward by pushing your hips back and letting your knees bend slightly. This is the same position as the barbell good morning (page 91). **2** Making sure to keep a neutral spine (or you'll injure your back), rotate your torso to the right as far as possible without moving your hips. You're trying to get the stick perpendicular to the floor. **3** Rotate back to the start and then the other way.

Figure 8 with Hold

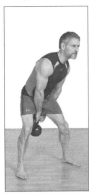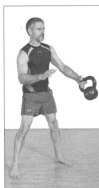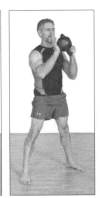

1 Stand with your feet about shoulder-width apart and hold a kettlebell in your right hand so that the pinky part is in the corner of the bell with your palm facing back. Push your hips back like you're going to do a swing. Keep your chest up, abs tight and back flat throughout this exercise. Your torso should naturally rotate toward the side the bell is moving. **2** Pass the bell between your legs to your left hand when the bell is behind your left knee. Your torso is rotated so the right shoulder is forward and the left back. **3** As the bell comes around your left knee, pop your hips and use your abs to stand up quickly into a forward-facing position, whipping the bell up. Don't use your arm to raise the bell, but do let your elbow bend and keep it close to your side. When you're standing tall, your left palm should be facing you and your right hand (palm outward) should come up at the same time to stop the bell from crashing into your chest or shoulder. **4** Push the bell out in front a little and rotate your left forearm so that the thumb points back to the right rear. Push your hips back and let the bell fall through your legs; your left shoulder is forward and your right is back. When it's behind your right knee, grab the bell with your right hand, letting the thumbs meet when the transfer occurs. **5** As the bell clears your right knee, whip it up by standing quickly again. This time, your right palm will be facing you and your left hand (palm outward) will act as a block.

Push the bell away from your body, take your hips back and repeat.

Slingshot

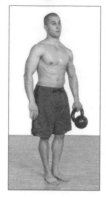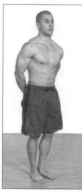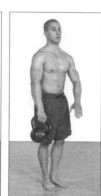

1 Stand with your feet together and hold a kettlebell with both hands in front of you. Your arms are hanging down, elbows straight. **2** Release the bell from one hand and move both arms behind you, one to each side. As you do the Slingshot, your hands will always face the rear. **3** Without moving your torso, bending at your ribs or twisting, use your free hand to grab the handle by the open corner and release the other hand. Keep your abs, glutes and lower back locked together throughout the movement to prevent your torso from bending or turning. **4** Bring both arms back to the front and transfer the bell to the other hand.

Continue passing the bell around your body, then switch directions.

PUSH-UPS

Bodyweight Push-Up

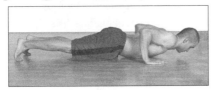

1 Place your hands on the floor directly under your shoulders. Step your feet straight back, shoulder-width apart, and lock out your hips. There should be a straight line from the base of your neck to your heels—do not lift your butt up or let it sag. **2** Slowly lower down, pointing your elbows to the rear. At the bottom position, your triceps and lats should touch. **3** Return to the top position, making sure you're actively pushing the floor away.

Knee Push-Up

Instead of having the balls of your feet on the floor, drop your knees to the floor but keep your back flat.

Incline Push-Up

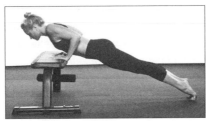

Place your hands on a sturdy surface that's higher than your feet. The steeper the incline, the easier the push-up. You can even put your hands on a wall and, as you get stronger, go lower and work off a bench or use aerobic steps and a riser to adjust the height.

Decline Push-Up

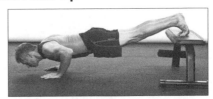

Place your feet on a sturdy surface that can't slide out from under you. This is much tougher than a regular push-up.

Triangle Push-Up

Instead of having your hands shoulder-width apart, bring them under your chest with your fingertips touching. These are tougher and hit the triceps much harder than a regular push-up.

Kettlebell Push-Up

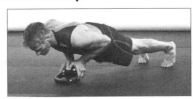

Place a kettlebell on the floor with the handle lying on the ground, facing forward. Place both hands on the bell, similar to the triangle push-up.

Spiderman Push-Up

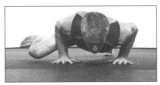

These require a lot more core and shoulder strength/stability than standard push-ups.

1 From a high plank, lower down for your push-up. As your body gets closer to the floor, pull one knee up toward your elbow on the outside of your body. Your inner thigh should be parallel to the floor. **2** As you drive away from the floor, return the leg to the start position.

On the next rep pull the other knee up.

Hindu Push-Up

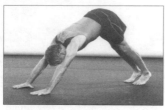

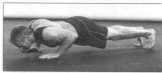

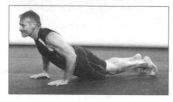

1 Assume a high plank and push your hips up and back. It's similar to Downward Dog in yoga. **2** Drop your chest down toward the floor and through your arms. Your chest should brush the ground or get as close as possible. **3** Push through until your chest faces forward and your pelvis is almost touching the floor; your back will arch. You're now almost in Upward Dog pose looking forward. **4** Push yourself straight up, returning to high plank, and drive your hips up and back.

T Push-Up

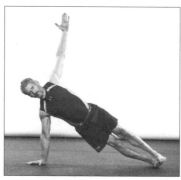

1 Assume a high plank. **2** Lower yourself toward the floor. **3** Push yourself away from the floor. As your elbows lock out, keep your left hand on the floor and rotate your entire body 90 degrees to the right. At the

same time, raise your right arm up so it's vertical. There should be a straight line from your right hand to your left hand and your right foot should be stacked on top of your left foot. If your feet are wider, roll your legs so that the inside of your right foot and the outside edge of your left is on the floor. **4** Rotate back to the high plank.

Switch sides.

Explosive Push-Up

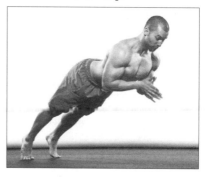

These are very difficult. Make sure you can do a regular push-up before you try these.

1 From a high plank, lower down for your push-up. **2** Keeping your feet on the floor and your spine neutral, explode your upper body up and clap your hands before quickly placing them back in the start position. Don't let your upper body move before your hips. As you land, absorb the force with your chest and stop yourself at the bottom push-up position.

PULL-UPS

Pull-Up

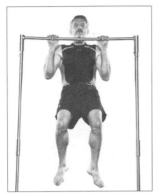

1 Hang from the bar with your hands in line with your shoulders or slightly wider and your palms facing forward. Pack your shoulders in their sockets and allow your legs and elbows to be slightly bent (this keeps tension through the upper body). **2** Contract all the muscles in your body and pull yourself up, thinking about bringing your elbows to your sides and your chin over the bar so it's parallel to the floor. Don't let your elbows flare out to the sides.

Lower yourself quickly but with control until you return to the start position. Pause then repeat. There should be no bouncing out of the descent and no leg swing.

Chin-Up

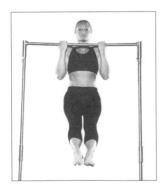

Hang from the bar with your palms facing you. This hits the biceps more than the back.

Inverted Row

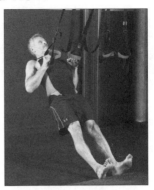

These hit the pull-up muscles at different angles, which will stimulate them to get stronger because the load is different and will help you to progress more quickly.

1 Set up a barbell so you can hang beneath it with your arms fully extended and torso parallel to the floor. Grab the bar with your hands about shoulder-width apart, palms facing away. **2** Pull your chest to the bar. Keep your elbows in, close to your body. Do as many as you can but not to failure.

Inverted Row with Rings

If you have access to gymnastics rings, you can perform inverted rows on them instead. They'll let you adjust the difficulty by changing your angle of inclination. The closer to parallel your body is to the floor, the harder the rows are. Try to keep your legs straight, but bend your knees slightly if you must.

PLYOMETRICS

Jumping Jacks

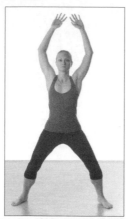

1 Stand with your feet together and palms facing your legs. **2** Quickly spread your legs to about 1.5 times shoulder-width apart (it should be comfortable without straining your knees) and at the same time bring your arms up the sides and overhead. Try to touch your hands. **3** Bring your feet back together and your arms to your sides. The hands and feet move together and never stop; this is a continuous movement.

Band Jumping Jacks

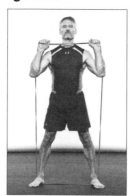

Step inside a light band with your feet about shoulder-width apart and hold the top corners of the band, palms facing forward. Jump your legs out wide and back to shoulder width as quickly as possible.

Jumping Jacks with Hammer Curl

1 Set up as above but turn your palms so they face each other. **2** As you jump out curl the band; as your feet come back to shoulder width straighten the arms. Keep your elbows at your sides and stay on the balls of your feet.

Squat Thrust

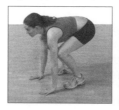 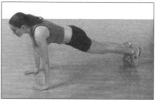

1 From a standing position, squat down and put your hands on the floor. **2** Drive your feet back so you're in a high plank. **3** Quickly pull your knees back under you, move back to your squat position and stand up.

Burpees

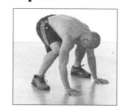 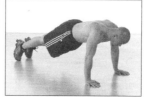

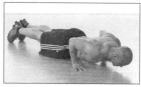

1 From a standing position, squat down and put your hands on the floor. **2** Drive your feet back so you're in a high plank. **3** Lower into a push-up. If you can't do a full push-up, do a partial push-up going halfway down, then as you fatigue start doing them on your knees. **4** Quickly pull your knees back under you, move back to your squat position and stand up.

Lateral Hop

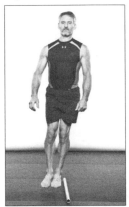

1 Stand tall with your feet together. **2** Keeping your torso forward, hop a few inches from side to side. The movement is from your hips and knees. Your feet come about an inch off the floor.

Squat Jump

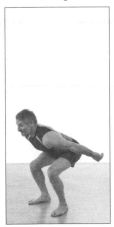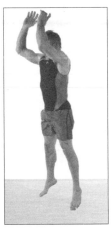

1 Stand with your feet about shoulder-width apart and pointed forward or turned out slightly. Staying flat-footed, pull yourself down as deep as you can go without leaning forward. Push your arms down hard behind you to give you extra power. **2** Explode upward but keep your toes on the floor as your hips fully extend (*note:* photo shows full squat jump). Once fully extended, sink your hips back and down onto your heels or as deep as you can go, letting your knees bend. Be graceful and soft—no jarring of the body.

Once you've mastered that, you can jump off the floor, keeping your legs fairly straight and your feet just a few inches off the floor. Use the same soft landing. Make contact with the balls of your feet first, then sink back onto your heels as your hips sink down, dropping back into a deep squat; repeat without pausing.

Weighted Jump Squat

Hold a kettlebell or dumbbell in your hands, drop into a quarter squat and jump as high as you can.

Jump Tuck

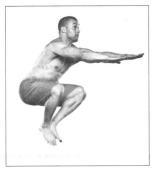

The jump tuck is very explosive since you have to violently pull both knees up as high as possible without the benefit of squatting to use the hamstrings and glutes.

1 Stand with your feet about shoulder-width apart and pointed forward or turned out slightly. **2** Contracting your hip flexors powerfully, bring your knees to your chest as quickly as possible, keeping your torso erect.

Land by quickly extending your hips and knees as you return to the ground. As soon as the balls of your feet touch the floor, pull your knees back up to your chest—don't allow your heels to contact the floor.

Mountain Climber

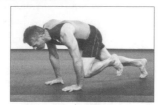

1 Assume a high plank with one knee tucked under you. You'll be supporting your weight with your upper body throughout the movement. Keep your elbows locked and hands shoulder-width apart. **2** Switch feet by quickly driving the tucked knee back and pulling the other knee under you. Your feet should not slide along the floor. The only time your feet touch the floor is the split second when one knee is up under you and the other leg is fully extended. As soon as you hit that position, move right through it and keep going.

Band around Hips Mountain Climber

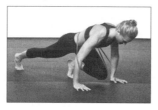

Place a resistance band around your hips and place one end in each hand as you set up for the mountain climber. This forces you to keep your core tighter.

Quad Press

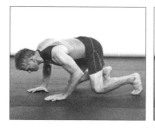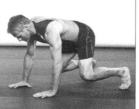

This is a very springy movement.

1 Start on hands and knees, with your hands a little wider than your shoulders, your knees slightly behind your hips, and your feet as wide as your hands. **2** Lift

your knees off the floor and straighten your elbows. Keep your back parallel to the floor. **3** Bend your elbows and knees and move toward the floor. **4** Keeping your back parallel to the floor, push away from the floor equally with both hands and feet. **5** When your elbows straighten out, quickly reverse the movement.

Quad Hop

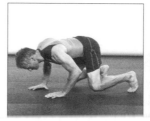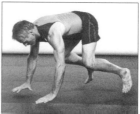

Because quad hops are so springy it may feel like you can pop off the floor. In the quad hop you do exactly that. This is much more difficult than the quad press so if you can't keep your back parallel to the floor on the quad press work on that before trying the quad hop.

1 Set up like the quad press. **2** Instead of pushing away from the floor with the hands and feet, explode up. **3** Land softly, absorbing your body weight into the chest, shoulders, feet, quads and glutes.

Remember: Your back needs to remain parallel to the floor.

Jump Rope

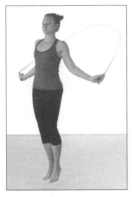

1 Hold a handle in each hand; keep your hands at about your waist line. The rope movement comes from the wrists, not the arms, so try to keep your elbows stationary. With the rope behind you, use your wrists to whip it over your head. As it comes down toward your feet, jump just high enough (an inch or so) to let the rope pass under your feet. The jumping is done with the calves and the balls of the feet; you'll never be flat-footed when jumping rope.

LEGS

Step-Up

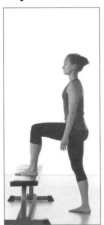

1 Stand in front of a sturdy box or other platform and step up onto it with both feet. Try to lift your knee and foot straight up. If you notice your foot moving to the outside or inside to clear the box, you'll need to work on

your hip flexibility.   **2** Step back with the same foot you started with.

Weighted Step-Up

Hold a kettlebell or dumbbell (either in goblet position or with your arm hanging along your side) and perform the step-up.

Step-Up with Reverse Lunge

Instead of bringing the other foot down next to the first (which would bring you to standing), move that foot behind you for a reverse lunge (page 114).

Step-Down

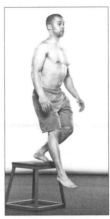

1 Stand on a step or box with both feet facing away from the box or step.   **2** Step one foot down to the floor then drive back up and return to a full standing position on the step.

Repeat with the other leg.

Weighted Step-Down

Hold a kettlebell or dumbbell (either in goblet position or with your arm hanging along your side) and perform the step-down.

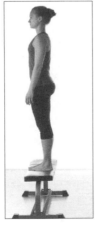

Machine Leg Press

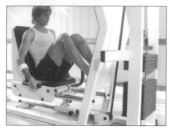

1 Using the leg press machine, load the weight or set the pin for the desired weight. Climb onto the sled and place your feet on the platform. Keep your lower back pressed into the back rest. **2** Keeping your knees pointed in the same direction as your toes, extend your hips and legs until your knees are straight, then slowly let them bend until the sled stops moving before pressing again.

Machine Leg Extension

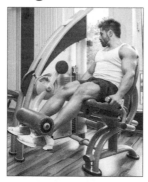

There are several types of machines for this. The most common is the bench with the padded pivoting arm at the end.

1 Sit on the bench with one or both shins under the pads. Hold onto the edge of the bench with both hands (or handles if your machine has them). **2** Contract your quads and straighten your knees. Hold briefly at the top before slowly lowering the legs by bending at the knees. Nothing moves above the knees.

Hamstring Curl with Stability Ball or Suspension System

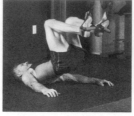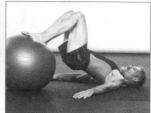

1 Lie on your back and place the backs of your calves on a stability ball or put your feet into the stirrups of a suspension trainer. Lift up your hips using your hamstrings and glutes and keep them up. Keep your lower back flat. **2** Bring your knees to your chest using your hamstrings and glutes. If using the ball, the bottom of your feet should be on the ball when your knees are fully bent.

1-Leg Hamstring Curl

To increase the difficulty, only use one leg on the ball or suspension trainer. Keep the other leg straight up in the air.

Squat & Kick

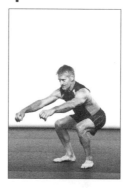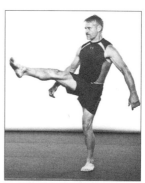

1 Perform a bodyweight squat. **2** As you return to standing, raise up one knee and kick straight ahead with the ball of your foot. **3** Bring your foot back to the floor where it started and descend into another squat. **4** Stand back up and kick out with your other foot.

Sklp

1 Stand with your arms by your sides. **2** Lift your right knee as high as possible and raise your left arm, bending the elbow until your hand is in front of the shoulder. As your right knee and left arm come up, rise up to the ball of your left foot and propel yourself forward a little. **3** Land on your right foot and lower your left hand. Hop forward a little, driving from your right foot, and bring your left knee and right arm up to skip on the other side.

Sprint

Becoming a good sprinter requires coaching as there are many intricacies of technique, which are beyond the scope of this book.

1 Stand with one foot a bit forward of the other, with each foot in line with its respective hip. Typically a right-handed person will have their right leg back. **2** Drive off the back leg as hard and fast as you can and pump your arms hard. **3** Run as fast as you can. Stay on the balls of your feet and keep your back flat. Look forward, not down.

Shuffle

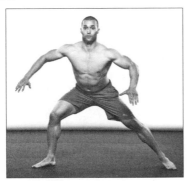

This is a sideways movement.

1 Stand with your feet about shoulder-width apart and hands by your sides. **2** Quickly bring your left foot next to your right foot. Just as quickly, slide your right foot away from your left foot so that your feet are shoulder-width apart again. Stay on the balls of your feet; they

barely come off the floor. Don't rotate your torso or bounce up and down—the movement is to the side only.

As you shuffle, incorporate your arms as well. As your left foot comes in, bring your arms up, crossing in front of your chest. Your arms stay crossed as your right foot moves out. When your left foot comes back in, your arms swing down and out to your sides. As your right foot moves out and lands, your arms are away from your body. As your left leg comes back in, your hands will come back up and cross again.

Carioca

This is another sideways movement.

1 Stand with your feet about shoulder-width apart. **2** Step with your left foot so it crosses in front of your right. **3** Step out with your right foot to shoulder width. **4** Now step your left foot behind your right foot. As you step, pivot your hip sharply to the left. **5** Step out with your right back to shoulder width, with hips facing straight ahead. **6** Step with your left foot in front of your right again. **7** Step out to shoulder width with your right. **8** Step behind with your left foot, pivoting your hips to the right.

ROPES

Ropes are a whole-body exercise and these are only a few of the many exercises that can be done with them. Most of them are undulating wave patterns—you're trying to make nice waves with the ropes. These teach you to use your body as a fluid unit. If the waves look bad, you're moving poorly. There's a lot of wrist, forearm and shoulder work as well as legs and core. However, I've never seen or heard of ropes causing or making worse any type of injury. They're very beneficial to the shoulders.

You'll need a 30-feet or longer rope that's 1.5" to 2" in diameter. You'll also need an anchor of some sort to loop the rope through or around. A round post works well, but it must be smooth or the rope will wear out quickly.

You have several choices for gripping the ropes.

Standard grip

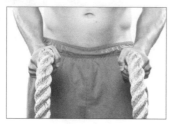

The ropes come into the palms through the thumb and forefinger. Your palms face each other.

Reverse grip

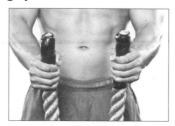

The ropes come into the palms from the bottom (i.e., pinky finger side of the hand). Your palms face each other.

Both ends of the rope in one hand

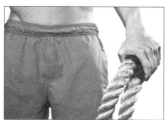

This is really tough on your grip, especially if you have small hands.

Double Wave

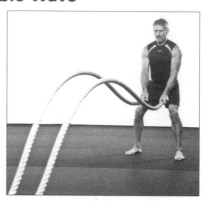

1 Stand facing the anchor with one end of the rope in each hand, hands at hip height, elbows bent and knees slightly bent. Your back should be neutral. **2** Sink down with your hips, bending your knees a little more, and stand up quickly, raising your forearms up and flexing your wrists. **3** Quickly drop down and let your forearms and wrists drop as well. Keep your elbows at your iliac crest (the bones at the top of your pelvis). **4** Rapidly reverse directions up and down, your arms moving with your legs. It's a pumping action.

Overhead Double Wave

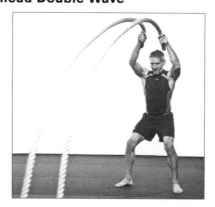

Instead of keeping your elbows in at your iliac crest, raise your hands over your head and let your elbows come up as well. This slows the pace but makes you move in a larger range of motion, moving the ropes higher and creating bigger waves.

Alternating Waves

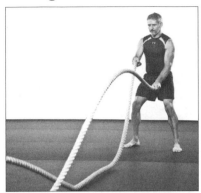

1 Start the same as the double wave (page 134). **2** Move one arm up and the other down in unison with the pumping action of the legs. There'll be more of a sideways movement of the hips rather than straight up and down. Make sure you're moving through the wrists—don't keep them locked in. The hand/arm movement is a drumming pattern.

Alternating Waves Slam

Let your hands come up higher, creating slower but bigger waves, and slam the rope hard into the ground.

In/Out Waves

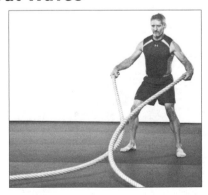

You'll feel this one in your lats. Make sure your wrists stay relaxed. Think of the original *Karate Kid* movie where Daniel-san is painting the fence.

1 Start the same as the double wave. **2** Separate your arms to your sides as you straighten your knees. **3** Quickly reverse your movement, bending your knees and bringing your arms in so that your wrists cross at your navel. **4** Rapidly reverse, moving your hands back out to the sides.

Outward Circles

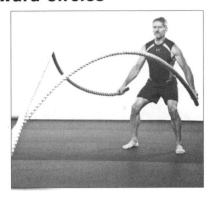

Your arms will be moving in opposite directions, each arm making a circle from outside to inside.

1 Start the same as the double wave. **2** As you stand up, quickly move your arms up to about shoulder height and out to your sides, down and around until each arm makes a circle. When the rope is shoulder high, you should be standing straight; when the rope is at its lowest point, your knees should be bent.

Alternating Outward Circle

Circle to one side and, at the halfway point, initiate a circle with the other side. You're 180 degrees out of synch. When one side is high, the other is low. Let your body flow with the movement.

Inward Circle

This is the exact opposite arm movement of the outward circle. Instead of going up, out and down, go down to the hips, up and out to the side, and peak at the shoulders so the wave of each part of the rope meets at the top instead of the bottom.

Alternating Inward Circle

This is the exact opposite of the alternating outward circle. One arm goes down, around and up to shoulder height, and the other arm does the same but 180 degrees out of synch with the first arm.

Slams

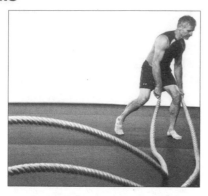

1 Start the same as the double wave (page 134). **2** Circle both hands (with the ropes) to the right and bring the ropes up higher than your head. As you begin the movement, lift your left heel and pivot through your hips and feet to the right. Your right toes should be out a little and both knees should be bent. **3** As the ropes start to pass over your head, pivot your feet so that your toes point to the left. **4** As the ropes continue to move in an arc and as you're pivoting, pull the ropes as hard as you can into the ground. When the ropes hit the ground, your right heel should be up with toes pointed left. Your left foot should be flat on the floor but toes out to the left a little. **5** Immediately circle the ropes in the opposite direction, pivoting your hips and feet to the right as the ropes come up and over. **6** Slam them into the ground and quickly reverse. Your left heel should be up with toes pointed left. Your right foot should be flat on the floor but toes out to the left a little.

MISCELLANEOUS

Tire Flip

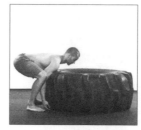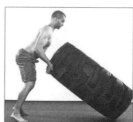
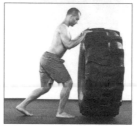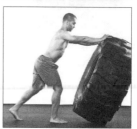

1 With the tire flat on the ground, squat down deeply with your chest touching the tire and your hips down. Hook your fingers underneath, preferably gripping the tread. **2** Lead with your shoulders and drive forward; extend your hips and stand. Use your legs, not your arms. As you stand, flip your hands from face up to palms forward. You may have to bump the tire with a knee during the transition phase for some added lift. Once you've switched your grip, drive through and push it over.

Sled Pull

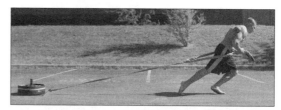

1 Grab the ropes of a sled and stand in front of it. **2** With your arms behind you at about hip level, stay tight and start walking forward. You'll have to dig in hard to pull heavy, driving with the balls of your feet. Don't try to pull with your arms. This really hits the quads hard!

Hand-Over-Hand Pull

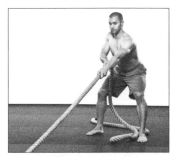

This can be done with a rope and sled or rope and several bells or other heavy objects.

1 Tie a heavy rope end to something heavy. Walk away from the weighted end until the rope is straight. Sit back into a squat stance with both hands on the rope, right hand closer to you than the left. **2** Pull with the right arm, rotating through your hips to the right. **3** Let go with your right and begin pulling with your left, rotating your hips to the left. While you're pulling, reach out with your right hand and grab the rope that's farther away from you. **4** Once you've finished pulling from the left, let go with your left and start to pull with your right, again rotating through your hips.

Continue switching hands and rotating until you've pulled the weight to you.

2-Handed Hand-Over-Hand Pull

You can also do a 2-handed pull, pulling to one side only. With both hands on the rope (right hand closer to you than the left) and left leg forward, pull the rope from the right side, rotating the hips right. Once you pull the weight in, straighten the rope back out and pull from the left side.

Wheelbarrow

Fill a wheelbarrow with heavy stuff and push it around.

Sledgehammer

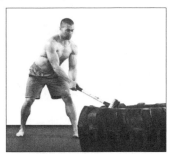

1 Stand with your feet about shoulder-width apart. Hold the sledgehammer to your lower right side; your right hand will be near the head of the sledgehammer, your left hand will be a few inches from the bottom of the handle. **2** Circle the sledgehammer down to the right a little then behind, up and over your right shoulder. **3** As the sledgehammer starts to come down, let your right hand slide down the handle so it ends up close to your left hand. At the same time sink your hips down and slam the sledgehammer into the tire. Be careful—It may bounce back! At the point of impact, tighten your grip or the sledgehammer will twist out of your hands.

You may now either do the right side again by sliding your right hand back up toward the head and moving the sledge to right rear again, or you can switch to a left-handed grip. Bring it to left rear, circling it back then up and over your left shoulder.

Sledgehammer with Staggered Stance

Occasionally you'll assume a staggered stance, with your right foot forward and left behind or vice versa. If your right foot is forward, you'll hit with a left-hand grip (left hand closer to the head); if your left foot is forward, you'll use a right-hand grip. The non-dominant grip will feel weird and you won't have nearly as much power or coordination for a while.

WARM-UPS

Spiderman Lunge with Rotation

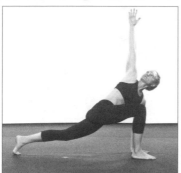

1 Step out into a lunge and place your hands on the floor inside your lead foot.   **2** Rotate your arm on the opposite side of the forward leg to the side and up. The movement should come from your hip and middle and upper back.   **3** Bring your arm back down, then lift both hands off the floor.   **4** Drive through your front leg and stand up, bringing your back leg forward.   **5** Continue to step through with what was the back leg into a lunge.   **6** Place your hands on the floor inside the front foot.   **7** Rotate your arm on the side opposite the front leg to the side and up.

Groiner

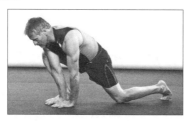

1 Start in a half kneeling position and place your hands on the floor inside the front foot.   **2** Maintaining neutral spine, rock forward, driving your knee past the toes, keeping your front foot flat on the floor.   **3** Rock back, maintaining neutral spine.

Do both sides.

If you can rock back far enough that the leg under you can straighten, you'll also feel a stretch in that

hamstring. However, don't round your lower back to get there.

Variation

If you have problems getting your hands on the floor, use a stool or post in front of you to hold on to, or place a yoga block on the floor and place your hands on it.

Hip Opener

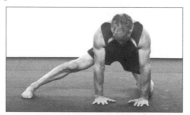

1 Assume the quadruped position, with your hands under your shoulders, arms straight and knees under your hips. Maintain a neutral spine, keeping your neck aligned with the rest of your spine.   **2** Extend one leg straight to the side with toes pointed forward, foot flat on the floor. The instep should be aligned with the knee of the leg under you.   **3** Keeping your back flat, rock back into your hips then rock forward. You should feel a stretch in the inner thigh of the outstretched leg and the hip flexor or the leg under you.

Do both sides.

Bootstrapper

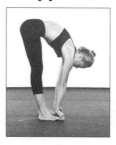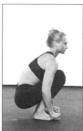

1 With your feet a little wider than your shoulders, bend over and grab your toes with your hands and stretch your hamstrings.   **2** Still holding your toes, pull your hips down and lift your chest up until you're in a deep squat with your lower back flat, not tucked under.   **3** Lift your hips, drop your head and chest, and straighten your knees to return to the start position.

Scapular Push-Up

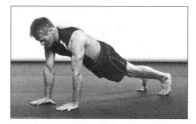

These strengthen the muscles that keep your shoulder blades pulled against your rib cage. Don't bend your elbows or allow your hips to move.

1 Assume a push-up position. You can do these on your knees if necessary. **2** Pinch your shoulder blades together. **3** Push the ground away, spreading your shoulder blades apart.

Walkout

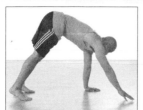 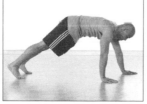

1 Stand with your feet hip-width apart. **2** Bend at the waist, trying to keep your knees straight, and put your hands flat on the floor in front of your feet. **3** Walk your hands out until you've reached at least a high plank position. Go farther if you can but don't let your hips sag. **4** Walk your hands back in. If you wish, you can stand up before walking your hands out again.

Variation

You can also add in a push-up when you reach the high plank position.

Half Kneeling Twist

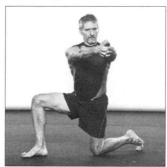

1 Assume the half kneeling position. Extend your arms at shoulder height, fingers interlaced as though you were holding a pistol. **2** Maintaining a tall spine, rotate mostly through the mid- and upper back as far to one side as you can. Pay attention to your posture and especially your front knee—don't let it fall in as your rotate. **3** Rotate back to center then to the other side, keeping the spine tall.

Dead Bug

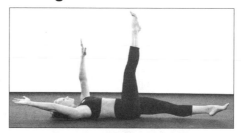

This core exercise works the glutes, quads, hip flexors and obliques as well as your shoulders and upper back.

1 Lie on the floor face up with your arms and legs extended. Try to keep both feet and both hands slightly off the floor at all times while keeping your torso and lower back pressed into the floor. **2** Slowly raise your right arm and left leg to the ceiling. Try to straighten your knee and point your toes up. Don't raise your head or shoulder when lifting the arm. **3** Slowly lower the arm and leg to just off the ground, then raise your left arm and right leg to the ceiling. **4** Slowly lower the arm and leg.

Quadruped Extension–Rotation

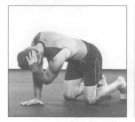 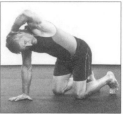

You should feel this between your shoulder blades and abs as they work to keep the lower back and hips from moving. If you feel this in your lower back, you're moving from your lower back instead of the middle and upper back.

1 Assume the quadruped position, with your hands under your shoulders, arms straight, and knees under your hips. Maintain a neutral spine, keeping your neck aligned with the rest of your spine. Place one hand on the back of your head.   **2** Rotating through your mid- and upper back, bring your elbow down and under toward your support elbow. Your head and eyes move with the elbow.   **3** Rotate back up and reverse the movement, extending as much as possible without losing neutral spine.

Wall Slide

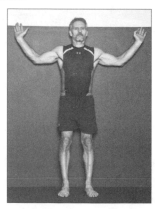

You should feel this between the shoulder blades.

1 Stand with your back to the wall and your feet 4 to 6 inches away from it. Your head, shoulder blades, lower back and hips should be touching the wall. If your lower back is excessively arched, either tuck your pelvis slightly

or move your feet a little farther from the wall. Hold your arms up, with elbows straight and hands out wider than your shoulders. The backs of your arms should touch the wall. You may already feel this in your lower back; don't let it arch.   **2** Keeping the backs of your arms against the wall and squeezing your shoulder blades together, pull your elbows down. Keep your head, shoulders, lower back and hips in contact with the wall.

Pause for a breath at the bottom. Only go as low as you can while keeping the backs of your arms on the wall.

Floor Slide

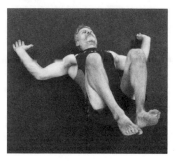

If you don't have a wall handy, do the wall slide on the floor.

1 Lie face up and bring your knees up, hips bent 90 degrees. Place your arms on the floor above your head wider than your shoulders. Keep the backs of your arms on the floor at all times.   **2** Squeeze your shoulder blades together as you pull your elbows down toward your sides. Keep your lower back on the floor! Hold at the bottom for 1 breath, then reverse the movement. Only go as low as you can while keeping the backs of your arms on the floor.

SELF-MYOFASCIAL RELEASE

Glutes

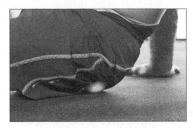

1 Sit on the floor and place the ball under your butt cheek. **2** Move your hip around, letting the ball work over tight muscles and trigger points. It won't be pleasant.

Do both sides.

Variation

You can also lie more sideways and hit the lateral part of your hip/glute (glutemedius).

Back of the Shoulders

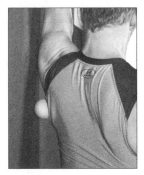

1 Stand against a wall and pin the ball between your upper trap and the wall. **2** Move your torso in a circular fashion so that the ball works all parts of the upper back, including the edges of the shoulder blade and lats.

Pecs

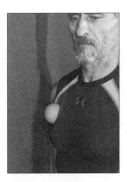

1 Face a wall and pin the ball between your upper chest and the wall. **2** Move your torso around so that the ball works all parts of your upper chest.

COOL-DOWNS

Hamstring Stretch

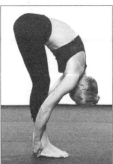

1 Stand tall with your feet and knees together. Sink your hips down and back as far as you can and place your fingers under your heels. If you can't reach your heels, go to the sides of your feet or toes. Keep your hips down. **2** Pull hard against your feet and lift your hips up high; keep pulling on your feet and lifting your hips. After 3 breaths, if you aren't able to fully straighten your knees, bend your hips slightly then lift them again. This should allow your legs to be straighter.

Kneeling Quad Stretch

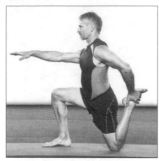

You may want a mat to pad the knee.

1 Get in a half kneeling position. Reach back with your hand and place the top of your foot in your palm. If your right knee is down, hold your right foot in your right hand.   **2** Maintaining a tall upright posture, slowly bring your rear foot toward its hip. Keep your torso and hips facing forward.   **3** Gently rock forward, exhale and hold, then rock back and inhale to increase the stretch.

Do both sides.

Variation

You may want to place a chair or bench in front of you and hold on with your other hand for balance. Ideally your front arm should be extended in front of you at shoulder height.

Down Dog

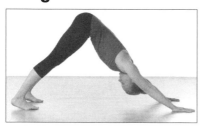

1 Start in high plank then drive your hips up and back, pushing back hard with your arms so that your head is between your arms but not hanging down; maintain a straight spine. From here, drive your heels toward the floor. You should feel a stretch in your calves and, if tight, your hamstrings and glutes. This, too, is an active pose so don't stay relaxed—push.

Down Dog for Ankles

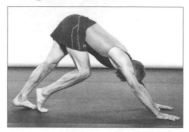

1 Start in high plank then drive your hips up and back, pushing with your arms.   **2** Drive one heel toward the floor; at the same time, flex the toes of the opposite foot. Your feet should be even and not move other than the heel lifting or moving toward the floor. If you're able to get your heel on the floor, move both feet back a little.   **3** Switch so you're now stretching the other foot and flexing the toes of the first foot.

Upward Dog

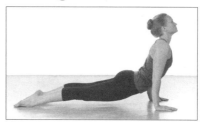

1 Lie on your stomach with your hands roughly beside your ribs and your fingers pointing forward; keep your elbows by your sides. Extend your legs behind you with the tops of your feet on the floor. Push the ground away, straightening your arms completely, so that only your palms and tops of your feet are on the floor. Reach your chest forward and up, keeping your shoulders down and away from your ears. Tilt your head back slightly, making sure not to crunch the back of your neck.

Standing Side Bend/Reach

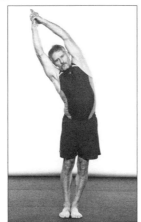

The goal is NOT to do a side bend but to actively push your hips as if you're doing a windmill (see page 101). You should feel a stretch in the lats on the same side as the hip pushing out. Inhale as you stand, exhale as you move to the side.

1 Stand with your feet together and bring your hands directly overhead, interlacing your fingers. The first finger of each hand points up.   **2** Push your hips to one side and reach up and out with the fingers to the opposite side. Exhale as you reach your end range and hold.   **3** Move through standing, pushing your hips to the other side while reaching with your fingers.

Cat/Cow

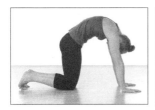 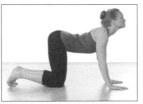

1 Place your hands and knees on the floor. Your hands are shoulder-width apart, right under your shoulders, and your knees are right under your hips so your thighs are vertical.   **2** Tuck your pelvis under, exhaling as you do so. Suck your navel to your spine and push the floor hard with your arms. Lift your upper back and feel your shoulder blades move apart. Tuck your chin to your chest. Hold for 3 breaths.   **3** Untuck your pelvis and chin at the same time, lifting both to the extreme opposite positions. Your hips are up, your lower back is curved down and your head is up. Continue to drive the ground away with your arms. You should feel your abs being stretched. Hold for 3 breaths and move back to cat.

Repeat 3 times.

Plow

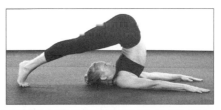

Be careful with this one. You may want a folded towel or yoga mat under your neck and shoulders. This stretches the upper back and, if you can get deep enough, the lower back as well.

1 Lie on the floor, exhale and bring your knees to your chest.   **2** Shift your weight onto your shoulders and extend your legs behind your head. Hold and breathe deeply into your belly for 3 to 4 breaths. When you extend your knees over your head you can try to touch the floor with your toes. However, you must be able to keep your knees straight; ideally your back is vertical and not rounded.   **3** Bring your knees back to your chest, shifting your weight to your entire back, and place your legs on the floor.

Pigeon

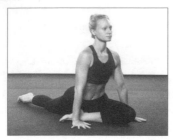

1 Sit on the floor with your shins under you, knees slightly apart. Slide one leg straight back and move the other leg out from under your thigh so that the outside of your shin is on the floor. Ideally your shin should be 90 degrees to the body with your foot in front of your body. However, most people don't have that much range of motion in their hips—don't force it. Think about pressing the hip of the bent leg toward the floor or use a yoga block under that hip and push into it. You may lie across the front leg or use your arms to support your upper body (easier). Once you're in position, hold for 4 to 5 seconds, taking 1 or 2 deep breaths, trying to relax and sink deeper into the pose. Do both sides.

PHOTO CREDITS

All photos © Rapt Productions except as noted below:

Page 80: Incline Bench Press © Mircea Netval/
shutterstock.com

Page 107: Front Raise © Philip Date/shutterstock.com

Page 107: Press-Down © Fotostorm/istockphoto.com

Page 108: Concentration Curl © Orange Line Media/
shutterstock.com

Page 110: Triceps Kickback © Ontario Incorporated/
shutterstock.com

Page 111: Dip © CEFutcher/istockphoto.com

Page 121: Back Extension on Ball © kenhurst/
istockphoto.com

Page 131: Machine Leg Press © david palau/
shutterstock.com

Page 132: Machine Leg Extension © Markus Gann/
shuterstock.com

Page 136: Sled Pull © Jessica Power

INDEX

INDEX OF EXERCISES